Gastric Sleeve Bariatric Cookbook

Tasty And Delicious Stage-by-Stage Recipes To Enhance Healthy Living And Long-Term Weight Loss Following Surgery

By: *Joseph L. Gonzalez*

TABLE OF CONTENTS

CHAPTER ONE: LIQUIDS STAGE 1 5
    1. Protein Hot Chocolate 5
    2. Peanut Butter Popsicles 6
    3. Creamy Chocolate Breakfast Shake 7
    4. BANANA & PEANUT BUTTER KEFIR PROTEIN SMOOTHIE 8
    5. Vegan Chocolate Milkshake 9
    6. Layer Fruit Smoothie 11
    7. Banana Yogurt Smoothie Recipe 12
    8. SAVORY AVOCADO TOMATO SMOOTHIE 13
    9. Easy Butternut Squash Soup 14
    10. CARROT GINGER SOUP 15

CHAPTER TOW: PUREES STAGE 2 17
    11. Watermelon Smoothie With Ginger and Lime 17
    12. Pina Colada Smoothie 18
    13. Mango Smoothie with Spinach and Banana 18
    14. Peveryes and Cinnamon Granola with Yogurt Panna Cotta 19
    15. Cinnamon, apple and ricotta cake 21
    16. DECADENT TOMATO BISQUE 22
    17. Green Pea Soup With Ham Recipe 23
    18. Savory Chicken Salad 25

CHAPTER THREE: SOFT FOODS STAGE 3 26
    19. Ricotta Banana Nut Bread Recipe 26
    20. cottage cheese banana bread (or muffins!) 28
    21. Soft Scrambled Eggs with Ricotta and Chives 30
    22. Egg Salad with Mustard 31
    23. CHEESY cauliflower casserole 32
    24. PASTA With Fresh Tomato Sauce and Ricotta 33
    25. AVOCADO and Black Bean Dip 34
    26. AVOCADO Tuna Salad Recipe 35
    27. GRILLED Salmon with Creamy Cucumber-Dill Salad 36
    28. CHICKEN Casserole Recipe 38
    29. EASY Baked Chicken 40
    30. BASIL Pesto Chicken Pasta 41
    31. Ground Chicken Shepherd's Pie 43
    32. STEAK-and-Potato Salad 46

CHAPTER FOUR: BREAKFAST 47

33. Pear, banana, oat and honey breakfast smoothie recipe 47
34. SUMMER Berry Parfait with Yogurt and Granola 48
35. PROTEIN porridge 49
36. Spinach Feta Omelet 50
37. SPINACH Parmesan Baked Eggs Recipe 52
38. SALMON and Eggs 53
39. Ricotta and Spinach Frittata With Mint 55
40. HEARTY Breakfast Burritos 56
41. TURKEY Hash Brown Breakfast Casserole 58

CHAPTER FIVE: VEGETARIAN 59

42. TAHINI banana date shakes 59
43. KEFIR GREEN SMOOTHIE 60
44. CHICKPEA Salad 61
45. Caprese Salad Recipe 62
46. STUFFED Jalapenos Pepper Recipe with Ricotta Cheese 64
47. PROTEIN Bowl (Vegan Buddha Bowl) 65
48. SPICY Mango, Black Bean & Avocado Tacos 68
49. Hummus Quesadillas! 69

CHAPTER SIX: SEAFOOD 71

50. NO-Mayo Mediterranean Tuna 71
51. Tuna Wraps 72
52. SHRIMP poke bowl recipe [sweet soy glaze + spicy mayonnaise] 73
53. GARLIC Shrimp with Quinoa 76
54. PESTO Shrimp and Broccoli Fettuccine + Weekly Menu 78
55. CREAMY GARLIC BUTTER TUSCAN SCALLOPS 79
56. HEAVENLY Halibut 81
57. SALSA salad 82
58. ONE-pan salmon with roast asparagus 83
59. ROASTED SALMON WITH YOGURT DILL SAUCE 84

CHAPTER SEVEN: POULTRY 86

60. CHICKEN SALAD WITH APPLES 86
61. CHICKEN CLUB MASON JAR SALADS 87
62. CHICKEN PESTO WRAPS 89
63. MEDITERRANEAN CHICKEN WRAP 91
64. Oven Chicken Kabobs 92
64. TERIYAKI CHICKEN STIR FRY 94
65. BAKED CHICKEN QUESADILLAS 96
57. LEMON PEPPER CHICKEN 98
58. SHEET PAN BALSAMIC CHICKEN & BRUSSEL SPROUTS 100

- 59. CREAMY MASHED CAULIFLOWER 102
- 60. THANKSGIVING LEFTOVER TORTILLA WRAP 103
- 61. GROUND TURKEY MEATLOAF WITH BROWN SUGAR GLAZE 105

CHAPTER EIGHT: PORK AND BEEF 107

- 62. CHEF'S SALAD RECIPE (REMEMBERING NAN) 107
- 63. CHEESY HAM & POTATO CASSEROLE 108
- 64. BAKED PORK CHOPS AND SAUERKRAUT 110
- 65. PULLED PORK SWEET POTATO SANDWICH 112
- 66. MEAT LOVER'S CROCK POT CHILI 113
- 67. BASIL MEATBALLS 115
- 68. UNSTUFFED PEPPERS 117
- 69. BUNLESS BURGER 118
- 70. MINI TACOS 120
- 72. ROAST BEEF WRAPS 121

CHAPTER NINE: DESSERT 122

- 73. FRESH PEVERY COBBLER 122
- 74. SWEDISH APPLE PIE (EASY CRUSTLESS APPLE PIE) 124
- 75. KETO PEANUT BUTTER BALLS 126
- 76. CANNOLI CHEESECAKE STUFFED STRAWBERRIES 128
- 77. NO-BAKE CHOCOLATE COCONUT SNOWBALLS 129
- 78. FRESH MANGO SALSA 131
- 79. SUN-DRIED TOMATO PESTO 132
- 80. PARMESAN CRISPS 133
- 81. Herb and Garlic Quinoa 134
- 82. Mashed Cauliflower and Potatoes 135

CHAPTER ONE: LIQUIDS STAGE 1

1. PROTEIN HOT CHOCOLATE

Prep Time: 5 minutes

Total Time: 5 minutes

Servings: 1

Ingredients

- ⅔ cup of milk + ⅓ cup of water use 2% or any dairy-free alternative
- I employ 1 scoop of protein powder with chocolate flavor whey.
- 1 tbsp cocoa powder
- 1 tbsp maple syrup
- 1 tsp vanilla extract
- Pinch of salt
- Mini marshmallows or whipped cream for topping

Instructions

Fill a small saucepan with all the ingredients except the toppings. Mix well until well blended. It's acceptable to have a few clumps. Heat the saucepan on medium for two to four minutes or until it is steaming and heated. To avoid burning and break up any clumps, whisk often. The hot chocolate will get a little thicker.
Once heated, transfer into a cup, garnish with whipped cream or miniature marshmallows, and serve immediately!

Nutrition

Calories: 255kcal | Carbohydrates: 33g | Protein: 26.5g | Fat: 3.8g | Cholesterol: 13mg | Sodium: 538mg | Potassium: 443mg | Fiber: 8g | Sugar: 20.5g | Calcium: 232mg | Iron: 0.8mg .

2. PEANUT BUTTER POPSICLES

Prep Time 5minutes

Total Time 5minutes

Yield 8 popsicles

Ingredients

- 1 cup of your preferred milk
- 1/3 cup of allergy-friendly

peanut butter or substitute

- A half-cup of coconut butter, 2 ripe bananas, or extra peanut butter
- 1/8 tsp salt
- sweeteners as needed, such as stevia, sugar, or pure maple syrup
- optional chocolate coating, listed below

Instructions

Process all ingredients for the popsicles in a blender until very smooth. Since the liquid will become less sweet when frozen, you want it overly sweet. The amount of sweetener you use will depend on your taste buds, the milk you choose, and the freshness of the bananas if used. Fill popsicle molds, then freeze.

Chocolate Coating: To make a sauce, either melt chocolate chips or mix 1/2 tbsp pure maple syrup or agave, 1 tbsp melted coconut oil, and 1 tbsp cacao or cocoa powder. Remove one popsicle from the freezer, coat it with sauce, transfer it to a wax paper-lined sheet, and then put it back in the freezer. Continue with the remaining popsicles.

3. CREAMY CHOCOLATE BREAKFAST SHAKE

PREP TIME 10 minutes

TOTAL TIME 10 minutes

Ingredients

- 2 ripe bananas that were cut and frozen before freezing
- 1/3 cup of frozen blueberries or strawberries
- 2-3 heaping Tbsp cocoa powder
- 2 tbsp salted almond butter
- 1 tbsp of optional flaxseed meal
- 1.5–2 cups of vanilla almond milk, unsweetened (substitute soy or coconut)
- 1 dash of agave nectar or stevia, depending on how sweet the bananas are
- 1/3 cup of ice
- 1 big handful of spinach (optional / not pictured here)

Instructions

Place all the ingredients in a blender and run it until everything is smooth.

Add extra cocoa powder to your smoothie if you like it more chocolaty. Add additional agave or stevia if that's how you want it sweeter. Add additional almond milk OR less ice if you'd like it thinner.

Nutrition (1 of 2 servings)

Serving: One shake has 312 calories, 48 grams of carbohydrates, 6.2 grams of protein, 1 gram of saturated fat, 14 grams of fat, and 0 grams of trans fat—cholesterol: 0 mg, Fiber: 7.5, Sugar: 27 g.

4. BANANA & PEANUT BUTTER KEFIR PROTEIN SMOOTHIE

prep time: 5 MINUTES

total time: 5 MINUTES

yield: 1-2 SERVINGS

INGREDIENTS

- 1 ½ cup ofs milk kefir
- 1 large frozen banana, halved
- 3 tbsp natural peanut butter
- 1 tbsp honey
- ½ tsp vanilla extract
- Pinch of ground cinnamon

INSTRUCTIONS

Fill the container of a strong blender (such as a Blendtec or Vitamix) with all your ingredients.

The process rapidly, pausing to scrape down the blender's edges if necessary.

Blend until smooth and well integrated, using all the ingredients. Blend again after tasting and adjust for sweetness or spices if necessary.

Transfer into a large tumbler or a pair of pint-sized glasses, then promptly serve.

If desired, drizzle with more peanut butter and a few chocolate chips.

NUTRITION INFORMATION:

Amount per serving: Calories: 330, total fat: 15g, saturated fat: 3g, trans fat: 0g, unsaturated fat: 10g, cholesterol: 8mg, sodium: 444mg, carbohydrates: 39g, fiber: 4g, sugar: 27g, protein: 15g.

---

5. VEGAN CHOCOLATE MILKSHAKE

PREP TIME 5minutes

TOTAL TIME 5minutes

SERVINGS 1 serving

INGREDIENTS

- Chocolate Milkshake
- Three peeled, chopped, and frozen bananas (overnight)
- 3/4 cup of rice milk (I used sweetened rice milk).
- 1 tbsp of Dutch-processed

cocoa powder

- 1 tsp of maple syrup

Toppings

- 1 tsp coconut oil
- 1 tsp maple syrup
- 1 tsp cocoa powder (dutch processed)
- soy whip
- 1/4 tsp shaved chocolate

INSTRUCTIONS

Whisk the cocoa powder, maple syrup, and coconut oil to make the chocolate sauce. Put aside.

Mix frozen bananas, rice milk, cocoa powder, and maple syrup in a high-speed blender for the chocolate milkshake. Blend until entirely smooth.

Transfer the milkshake into a tall glass, then top with shaved chocolate, soy whip, and homemade chocolate sauce. Have fun!

NUTRITION

Calories: 498kcal, Carbohydrates: 113g, Protein: 5g, Fat: 7g, Sodium: 74mg, Potassium: 1343mg, Fiber: 11g, Sugar: 60g, Vitamin A: 225IU, Vitamin C: 30.8mg, Calcium: 36mg, Iron: 1.6mg .

6. LAYER FRUIT SMOOTHIE

Prep time 1 hour

Total time: 1 hour

Serves: 3-4

Ingredients

- ½ cup of Almond Breeze almond milk Vanilla
- ¼ cup of + 2 tbsp almond butter
- ½ frozen banana
- 1 tbsp cocoa powder
- 2 soft Medjool dates, pitted
- handful of ice
- Middle Layer: Banana Vanilla
- 1 cup of vanilla Almond Breeze almond milk
- 1½ frozen bananas
- 2 soft Medjool dates, pitted
- 1 scraped vanilla bean or one Tsp of pure vanilla essence
- handful of ice
- Top Layer: Red Berry
- 1 cup of strawberries, frozen
- 1 cup of frozen raspberries
- 1 cup of Almond Breeze almond milk Vanilla
- Chocolate chips for garnish, optional

Instructions

Mix the dates, cocoa powder, banana, almond milk, and almond butter in a blender to make the bottom layer. Blend until completely pureed and the dates are smooth—pulse after adding the ice. Transfer into three or four smaller glasses and place in the freezer for half an hour.

Make the center layer in a blender, combining the almond milk, dates, bananas, and vanilla; process until smooth. Pulse after adding the ice. After adding this layer to the smoothies, freeze for half an hour.

To Make the upper layer, put the almond milk, strawberries, and raspberries in a blender and process until smooth. It will be a very thick coating. Spoon the last layer atop the smoothies after removing the glasses from the freezer. If desired, top with chocolate chips.

Since the bottom two layers are not frozen, it should take five to ten minutes for them to thaw and become spoonable-like consistency. Present and savor.

7. BANANA YOGURT SMOOTHIE RECIPE

Prep Time5 Minutes

Total Time5 Minutes

Serves2

Ingredients

- 2 bananas
- 1 cup of milk
- ½ cup of plain yogurt
- 1 Tbsp honey
- 1 tsp vanilla essence

Instructions

Blend bananas, yogurt, milk, honey, and vanilla.

Blitz till mixable.

Present and enjoy.

Nutritional Data

Amount per serving:36.9g, carbohydrates, 2.5g dietary fiber, 26.5g sugars, 11 mg cholesterol, 82 mg sodium, 7.1g protein, 2.9g total fat, 1.8g saturated fat, and 0g trans fat.

8. SAVORY AVOCADO TOMATO SMOOTHIE

Prep time: 5 minutes

Total time: 10 minutes

What You'll Need

- One large avocado, seeded and sliced
- ½ cup of chicken or vegetable broth
- ½ Red Sun Farms Roma Tomato
- ½ cup of whole milk or coconut milk
- 1 tbsp lime juice
- 1 scoop of protein powder that is unflavored and unsweetened (whey, rice, fermented soy, or egg are optional).
- ¼ cup of sliced white onions, around one inch in size
- 1 tbsp of raw cilantro
- Sea salt and black pepper as needed

Directions

In a blender, mix all the ingredients and process until smooth. Serve right away.

9. EASY BUTTERNUT SQUASH SOUP

Prep Time: 10 minutes

Cook Time: 25 minutes

Total Time: 35 minutes

Ingredients

- ½ Tbsp. olive oil
- 2 minced garlic cloves
- 1 onion diced
- 1 butternut squash, chopped into cubes after peeling.
- 32 ounces of vegetable broth
- 1-2 tsp. salt

Instructions

In a Dutch oven, warm the olive oil over medium heat. Add the garlic and onion. Simmer for about five minutes or until the food is soft.

Add the cubed butternut squash and the veggie broth. After raising to a boil, decrease heat, cover, and simmer until squash is cooked 15 to 20 minutes.

Pour all the contents of the pot. I use my Vitamix blender carefully into the blender. Put some salt in.

Blend till smooth, using care. Garnish with thyme and serve in dishes. Have fun!

Nutrition

135 kcal of calories, 24g of carbohydrates, 4g of fat, 1g of saturated fat, 1 mg of cholesterol, 884 mg of sodium, 3 grams of fiber, and 4 grams of sugar.

10. CARROT GINGER SOUP

PREP: 30minutes

COOK: 30minutes

TOTAL: 1hour

SERVINGS: 4 servings

INGREDIENTS

- 2 tbsp avocado oil or olive oil
- 1 medium onion, diced
- 3 cloves garlic, minced
- 3 tsp of finely chopped or minced ginger
- 2 pounds carrots, peeled and chopped
- 4 cups of vegetable broth
- 1 bay leaf
- 1 tsp cinnamon
- 1 tsp salt

Topping options include toasted pine nuts, cilantro, coconut cream, and crispy shallots.

INSTRUCTIONS

Stirring constantly, warm the oil in a big pot. Add the onions and boil for one to two minutes or until they are translucent.
Pour in the garlic and ginger and stir for a minute more.

Stir everything together in the saucepan after adding the diced carrots. Cook for five minutes, stirring often.

Add the salt, bay leaf, cinnamon, and broth to the pot. When it boils, reduce it to a medium simmer and cover. Cook the carrots for 20-30 minutes, or before a fork is put into them, it yields mush.

Remove the bay leaf once the heat has been turned off. Combine the soup with an immersion blender or move it to a powerful one. In a blender, puree the soup until it's smooth.

Divide the soup in half between every bowl. Toppings: Top with crispy shallots, cilantro, and a tbsp of coconut cream if desired.

NUTRITION

186KCAL, 29G of carbohydrates, 3G of protein, 8G of fat, 1680MG of sodium, 799MG of potassium, 7G of fiber, 14G of sugar, 92MG of calcium, and 1MG of iron.

CHAPTER TWO: PUREES STAGE 2

11. WATERMELON SMOOTHIE WITH GINGER AND LIME

Prep Time 15 minutes

Total Time 15 minutes

Servings 4 People

Ingredients

- 3 Cup of Watermelon - Cut into 2" cubes
- 1/2 Tsp Ginger - Juice from fresh ginger root. Vary as need
- 1/2a Tsp of lime juice or lemon juice
- 1/4 Tsp Himalayan Pink Salt - Or as needed
- 2 Tbsp Mint Leaves - Fresh Leaves. Vary as need
- Or, as needed, use 1/8 tsp of cayenne pepper.

Instructions

Watermelon should be sliced into 2-inch chunks and added to a blender. Add the ginger juice, cayenne pepper, lemon or lime juice, mint leaves, and salt.

Blend quickly. Taste and modify the flavor as necessary, adding more salt for electrolytes, watermelon for sweetness, or mint for a more robust herb flavor.

Distribute among the serving glasses and savor. Garnish with fresh mint, if desired. Though leftovers can be stored covered in the refrigerator for up to two days, they are best when fresh. To make yourself feel better in the afternoon, freeze leftovers in popsicle molds or ice cube pans.

12. PINA COLADA SMOOTHIE

PREP TIME 5 mins

TOTAL TIME: 5 mins

SERVINGS 1 smoothie

INGREDIENTS

- 1/2 frozen banana
- 1/2 cup of frozen pineapple chunks
- 1/3 cup of pineapple or pina colada juice
- 1/4 cup of coconut milk
- a handful of ice cubes

INSTRUCTIONS

In a blender, mix all ingredients. Blend for one minute or until smooth. Serve right away.

13. MANGO SMOOTHIE WITH SPINACH AND BANANA

TOTAL: 5minutes

SERVINGS: 1 (large) smoothie

Ingredients

- Frozen mango chunks, about 10 ounces (1 1/2 cups)

- 1 ripe banana cut into chunks
- 1 cup of packed baby spinach leaves
- 3/4 cup of unsweetened almond milk

Instructions

Put the frozen mango, banana, spinach, and almond milk into your blender.
Process till smooth. Savor right now.

Nutrition

Serving: 1smoothiecalories: 299kcal, carbohydrates: 72g, protein: 1g, fat: 2g, saturated fat: 2g, fiber: 8g sugar: 54g.

14. PEVERYES AND CINNAMON GRANOLA WITH YOGURT PANNA COTTA

Prep Time: 15 mins

Cook Time: 10 mins

Total Time: 25 mins

Ingredients
Peveryes and Vanilla Yogurt Panna Cotta:

- 1 packet containing 1/4 Ounces (3 tbsp) of flavorless gelatin powder
- 1 ½ cup of heavy (whipping) cream, divided
- ⅓ cup of sugar, grated
- 1 pinch kosher salt
- 2 cups (17.6 Ounces/500 gm) of plain, thick Greek yogurt
- 1 tsp vanilla extract

- 2 canned slices every can (15 Ounces every), drained

Small Batch Cinnamon Granola:

- 1 cup of rolled oats
- 1 tbsp of powdered cinnamon
- 1 tbsp honey
- ¼ cup of whole or halved almonds
- 1 pinch of sea salt

Instructions

Peveryes and Vanilla Yogurt Panna Cotta:

Spread the gelatin on a small plate with 1/4 cup of water and let it soften for about five minutes.

Meanwhile, in a small saucepan, bring one cup of cream, sugar, and salt to a boil, stirring until the sugar dissolves. Take off the heat and mix in the gelatin.

Whisk together yogurt and the remaining 1/2 cup of cream in a bowl. Mix in vanilla and gelatine mixture. Distribute evenly among eight serving plates and place in the refrigerator to solidify, which might take up to overnight.

Small Batch Cinnamon Granola:

Set oven temperature to 350°F.

After spreading out on a baking sheet, bake the oats for ten minutes.

Stir in the salt, honey, almonds, and cinnamon. After mixing well, put the mixture back in the oven. Bake for a Another 15 to 20 minutes.

Let it cool.

Assembly:

Best Yogurt Panna Cotta with Granola and Peveryes.

15. CINNAMON, APPLE AND RICOTTA CAKE

Prep 30m

Cook 1h 20m

Serves 12

Ingredients (16)

- 3 Granny Smith apples
- 1 tbsp honey
- 1 1/2 cups of (225g) self-raising flour
- 1/2 cup of (60g) almond meal
- 1 cup of (220g) caster sugar
- 1/2 cup of (85g) cornmeal (polenta)
- 1 tsp baking powder
- 2 tsp ground cinnamon
- 2 tsp finely grated orange rind
- 125g butter, melted
- 2 Coles Brand Australian Free Range Eggs, lightly whisked
- 1/2 cup of (125ml) milk
- 500g fresh firm ricotta
- 2 tbsp brown sugar
- Crème fraîche, to serve
- Honey, extra, to serve

Method

Set oven temperature to 160°C. Grease a 20cm (base measurement) springform pan, then line the side and base with baking paper.

Cut two of the apples thinly crosswise. Chop the remaining apple into pieces. Chop finely. Put aside. Line the bottom of the prepared pan with half of the sliced apple. Pour over the honey.

Mix the flour, almond meal, caster sugar, cornmeal, baking powder, half of the cinnamon, and half of the orange rind in a large basin. Stir in the diced apple after adding it. Stir the butter, egg, milk, and half of the ricotta cheese.

In another basin, stir the brown sugar, orange peel, and remaining cinnamon with the ricotTA.

After the pan is ready, spoon half the batter over the apple. Make the surface smooth. Place the leftover apple slices on top of the batter. Smooth the apple's surface after Adding the ricotta mixture. Cover with the leftover batter, making sure the surface is smooth. A bamboo skewer put into the center should come out clean after baking for one hour and twenty minutes. Place aside in pan to cool thoroughly.

Place the cake onto a platter for serving. Cut into wedges and serve with more honey poured over crème fraîche.

16. DECADENT TOMATO BISQUE

Ready In: 7mins

Serves: 6

INGREDIENTS

- 2(14 1/2 ounce) cans of stewed tomatoes, coarsely chopped
- 1cup of whipping cream
- 1tsp dried basil (or more, as needed)

DIRECTIONS

Put the stewed tomatoes into a pot.

Before rising to a boil, reduce the heat and simmer.

Add cream and stir.

Add basil and stir.

And voilà!

17. GREEN PEA SOUP WITH HAM RECIPE

Prep Time: 0 minutes

Cook Time: 15 minutes

Yield: 4–5 service

INGREDIENTS

- 1 Tbsp. olive oil
- 1 Tbsp. butter
- 1 cup of carrot matchsticks*, roughly chopped
- 1 small onion, chopped
- 7 Ounces smoked ham, finely chopped
- 32 Ounces frozen green peas
- 2 cloves garlic, minced
- 3 cups of low-sodium chicken broth
- 1/2 tsp. salt
- 1/4 tsp. dry thyme leaves
- 1/8 tsp. black pepper

INSTRUCTIONS

Melt butter olive oil in a big saucepan (Dutch oven set over medium-high heat). To the saucepan, add the ham, carrot, and onion. After covering the pot, turn down the heat to medium.

Place the frozen peas in a big bowl safe to microwave—heat for four to six minutes on high.

In the meantime, stir-fry the garlic in the saucepan for 30 seconds. Next, add the salt, black pepper, and thyme to the chicken broth. After stirring, cover. Elevate the temperature to high and let the soup boil. Simmer the heat now.

Using a ladle, spoon some stock over the heated peas once the broth has simmered. Puree the pea mixture with an immersion blender until it's very smooth. Alternatively, mix this in batches. Refit the pot's lid, then boil the soup until the carrots are soft.

Stir the mushy peas after transferring them into the broth. Warm up thoroughly. Add extra broth to your soup if you want it thinner.

NUTRITION

Total fat 12.9g, cholesterol 54.2mg, sodium 560.1mg, total carbohydrate 39.4g, sugars 12.3g, protein 30.5g, vitamin A 493.7µg, vitamin C 26.1mg.

18. SAVORY CHICKEN SALAD

Prep Time 15minutes

Cook Time 0minutes

Total Time 15minutes

Servings: 8 Cup of

Ingredients

- 1 ½ lb cooked chicken
- ½ cup of finely diced celery
- ½ cup of chopped pecans
- 2 tbsp finely diced red onion
- 1 tbsp Dijon mustard
- 2 tbsp dill or sweet relish
- 1 ¼ cup ofs mayonnaise
- Optional: sugar or sugar substitute

Instructions

Chicken, celery, pecans, red onion, dijon mustard, relish, and mayonnaise should all be mixed in a big bowl. Combine the soup with an immersion blender or move it to a powerful one. Use a hand mixer until thoroughly blended. Add your preferred seasonings and salt and pepper if your chicken isn't seasoned (unlike the rotisserie chicken in the video). Refer to the Note.
Until you're ready to serve, please keep it in the refrigerator in an airtight container.

Nutrition

Serving: 1cup of | calories: 275kcal | Carbohydrates: 5g | protein: 22g | fat: 18g | cholesterol: 69mg | sodium: 379mg | potassium: 256mg | fiber: 1g | sugar: 2g | vitamin a: 93iu | vitamin c: 0.5mg | calcium: 21mg | iron: 1mg .

CHAPTER THREE: SOFT FOODS STAGE 3

19. RICOTTA BANANA NUT BREAD RECIPE

Prep Time:15MINUTES

Cook Time:1HOUR

Total Time:1HOUR 15MINUTES

Ingredients

- A half-cup of virgin olive oil, pure (melted butter or coconut oil work well as substitutes)
- 1/2 cup of white granulated sugar
- 1/3 cup of brown sugar
- 2 large organic eggs
- 2 vanilla bean seeds or two tsp of Essence
- 1/2 a cup full-fat ricotta cheese
- 1 tbsp heavy cream
- 1 1/2 cup of all-purpose flour
- 1 tsp of baking soda
- 1/2-tsp of baking powder
- 1 dash of sea salt
- 3/4 cup of coarsely chopped candied walnuts + a few more for garnish

- 2 bananas – diced

Instructions

Set the oven to 350°F.

The creamy texture is achieved by whisking sugar and melted butter or olive oil together in a medium-sized basin.

Whisk in the heavy cream, ricotta cheese, and vanilla extract until well-mixed. Add the eggs and whisk again once the mixture is smooth. Add the walnuts and bananas, tossing gently to coat.

Combine baking powder, flour, soda, and sea salt in a big Dish. Pour the wet ingredients into the well that you made in the center.

Gently mix all the ingredients using a spatula.

After lightly greasing the loaf pan with butter or oil, pour the ingredients into it.

As a garnish, add a few walnuts on top.

Set the oven's temperature to 350 degrees. When a toothpick in the center comes out clean, bake for one hour. Place it on a cooling rack after transferring it to a wooden cutting board.

Nutrition

calories (422 kcal), 21g fat, 51mg cholesterol, 217mg sodium, 203mg potassium, 51g carbs, 7g protein, 2g fiber, 28g sugar, 69 mg calcium, and 2mg iron.

20. COTTAGE CHEESE BANANA BREAD (OR MUFFINS!)

Total Time: 65 minutes

Yield: 10 slices

INGREDIENTS

- 1 heaping cup of mashed ripe banana (about 3 small to medium bananas)
- 1/2 a cup of either thinly packed brown sugar or raw maple syrup
- 1/3 cup of avocado oil
- 2 eggs
- 2/3 cup of cottage cheese
- 1/4 cup of hemp hearts
- 1 tsp vanilla
- 3/4 cup of white whole wheat/all-purpose flour
- 1 tsp baking soda
- 1 tsp cinnamon
- 1/2 tsp salt
- 1/2 cup of mix-ins of choice like walnuts, chocolate chunks, pecans, pumpkin seeds, coconut or dried cranberries

INSTRUCTIONS

Oven prep: Set the temperature to 325 degrees. Standard-sized loaf pans measuring nine by 5 inches should be greased with butter or nonstick baking spray and lightly dusted with flour to remove excess. Place the ready pan aside. If you use a glass loaf pan, be aware it will take longer to bake; I like using a metal loaf pan.

Wet ingredients: Mash the bananas in a big bowl until they are "liquid"; some lumps may occur, but that's acceptable. Add the oil and brown sugar and whisk. Whisk the eggs, cottage cheese, hemp hearts, and vanilla essence well.

Dry ingredients: Place the flour, baking soda, salt, and cinnamon in the same bowl. The dry components should be JUST mixed with the liquid mixture after being folded using a silicone spatula. An overmixed loaf turns out to be rougher and more dense. Stir in any add-ins.

Bake: Transfer the mixture to the ready pan. You may carefully press a sliced banana or a handful of chocolate bits onto the top of the bread. When a toothpick inserted into the center of the bread comes out clean, bake for 55 to 60 minutes.

Cool: After letting the loaf cool in the pan for fifteen minutes, release it by slicing it with a knife along its edge. Please remove the loaf and let it cool down for a few more minutes on a cooling rack (I know it's impossible).

Have fun: Cut and present! My favorite is covered with peanut butter, but STRAIGHT UP is also delicious, as well as butter, almond butter, and honey.

Nutrition

Total fat 11.1g, cholesterol 39mg, sodium 305.6mg, total carbohydrate 32.5g, dietary fiber 3.2g, sugars 13.3g, protein 7.1g, vitamin A 27µg, vitamin C 2.1mg, calcium 52.2mg, iron 1.4mg.

21. SOFT SCRAMBLED EGGS WITH RICOTTA AND CHIVES

PREP TIME: 5MINUTES

COOK TIME: 5MINUTES

TOTAL TIME: 10 MINUTES

SERVINGS: 1 SERVING

Ingredients

- 1 tbsp butter
- 2 tsp full-milk ricotta cheese
- As needed, add salt and Pepper.
- Taste and add black Pepper
- Butter toast for serving is optional, as is chopped soft, fresh herbs like dill, basil
- parsley, or chives.

Instructions

Pour the cracked eggs into a small basin.

Beat the eggs thoroughly until light and airy, with no white or yolk streaks. To make things easier, I like to use an immersion blender.

Melt the butter in a little pan set over medium-low heat. Pour in the eggs and slowly make giant curds by lifting and folding them with a rubber spatula as you go.

Remove from the fire when the eggs are almost set, then stir in the ricotta, salt, and Pepper.

Place the eggs onto a dish. If preferred, garnish with herbs and serve right away on buttered bread.

Nutrition

Calories: 278kcal | Carbohydrates: 2g | Protein: 15g | Fat: 24g Cholesterol: 373mg | Sodium: 240mg | Potassium: 156mg | Sugar: 0.4g | Vitamin A: 959IU | Calcium: 115mg | Iron: 2mg.

22. EGG SALAD WITH MUSTARD

Prep Time: 5 mins

Cook Time: 5 mins

Additional Time: 20 mins

Total Time: 30 mins

Servings: 3

Yield: 3 servings

Ingredients

- 6 large eggs
- 5 green onions, white parts only, minced
- ⅓ cup of mayonnaise
- 2 tbsp dill pickle relish
- 2 tbsp chopped fresh parsley
- ½ tbsp sweet hot mustard
- ½ tbsp spicy brown mustard

Directions

After placing the eggs in a heavy pot, cover the top of the pot with water by approximately an inch. Bring over medium-high heat to a rolling boil. Please take off the heat source and let it sit for fifteen minutes. Put in a five-minute ice bath. Take the shells off.

Process eggs in a food processor or by hand until the required consistency is revealed.

Whisk together eggs, green onions, mayonnaise, relish, parsley, spicy brown mustard, and sweet hot mustard in a bowl.

23. CHEESY CAULIFLOWER CASSEROLE

Prep Time: 15 minutes

Cook Time: 40 minutes

Total Time: 55 minutes

Yield: 6 servings

ingredients

- Cut into florets 1 big head of cauliflower.
- 2 tbsp butter
- 2 tbsp flour
- 1 cup of milk
- 1 cup of shredded cheddar cheese
- Freshly ground Pepper

instructions

Steam cauliflower for ten minutes or until the florets are soft.

Butter a casserole and heat the oven to 400.

Mix in flour until thoroughly mixed.

Add milk, whisk, and boil until just thickened. Turn off the heat and blend in the cheese.

After spreading the cauliflower in the casserole, cover it with the cheese sauce. Sprinkle some pepper on top.

After 30 minutes of baking, gently cool and serve.

Nutrition

Total Fat 11.3g, Saturated Fat 6.5g, Trans Fat 0.2g, Cholesterol 32.1mg, Sodium 358.1mg, Total, Carbohydrate 15.7g, Dietary Fiber 0.8g, Sugars 11.9g, Protein 6.6g.

24. PASTA WITH FRESH TOMATO SAUCE AND RICOTTA

Total Time: 30 minutes

Yield:4 to 6 servings

INGREDIENTS

- 1pound dried pasta, such as farfalle or penne
- Salt and Pepper
- 2tbsp butter, softened
- Crushed red Pepper (optional)
- 2½ cups of Quick Fresh Tomato Sauce, warm (see recipe)
- 6ounces ultra-fresh ricotta, at room temperature
- Grated pecorino
- Basil leaves, for garnish
- Add to Your Grocery List

PREPARATION

Keep the pasta fairly al dente when cooking it in a big saucepan of well-salted water.

Heat a broad, deep skillet with butter over medium heat. If using, pasta that has been drained should be added to the pan along with salt, Pepper, and crushed red Pepper.

Using enough liquid for a light coating, gradually add the tomato sauce and stir to coat the pasta (you may not need to use all 2½ cups).

Place the spaghetti in a heated serving bowl and sprinkle some ricotta cheese. Add some pecorino cheese and some torn basil leaves as garnish.

25. AVOCADO AND BLACK BEAN DIP

Prep Time:10 mins

Cook Time:1 mins

Total Time:11 mins

Servings:4

Yield:4 servings

Ingredients

- 1 avocado - peeled, pitted, and mashed
- ½ (15 ounces) can of rinsed and drained black beans
- 1 tbsp lime juice
- one finely chopped garlic clove, or extra as needed
- ⅓ cup of shredded Cheddar cheese
- 1 pinch of sea salt as needed

Directions

Place the avocado, black beans, lime juice, and garlic in a safe microwave bowl. Add a little cheddar cheese on top.

Melt cheese in the microwave on high for 1 minute or until it's melted. If preferred, season with sea salt.

26. AVOCADO TUNA SALAD RECIPE

Prep Time: 10 minutes

Total Time: 10 minutes

Servings: 6 as a side salad

Ingredients

- 3 little cans, 15 ounces of drained and flaked tuna in oil
- 1 English cucumber, sliced
- Peel, pit, and slice two big or three medium avocados
- Thinly slice 1 small or medium red onion.
- 1/4 cup of cilantro, (1/2 of a small bunch)
- 2 Tbsp lemon juice, freshly squeezed
- 2 tbsp extra virgin olive oil
- 1 tsp sea salt, or as needed
- 1/8 tsp of black Pepper

Instructions

Place the sliced avocado, sliced cucumber, red onion, drained tuna, and 1/4 cup of cilantro in a large salad dish.

Add 2 tablespoons lemon juice, 1 teaspoon salt, tablespoons olive oil, and 1/8 teaspoon black pepper (or season to taste) to the salad components. Combine and proceed to serve.

27. GRILLED SALMON WITH CREAMY CUCUMBER-DILL SALAD

Cook Time: 10 Minutes

Total Time: 30 Minutes

Servings: 4

INGREDIENTS
FOR THE SALMON

- 4 (6-ounces) salmon fillets, skin on
- 1 tbsp extra virgin olive oil
- ¾ tsp kosher salt
- ½ tsp freshly ground black Pepper

FOR THE CREAMY CUCUMBER-DILL SALAD

- 1 English cucumber (also called hothouse cucumber)
- One little red onion yields ⅓ cup of thinly sliced onion.
- ½ tsp salt
- ¼ cup of + 2 tbsp sour cream
- 3 tbsp good-quality mayonnaise, such as Duke's or Hellmann's
- 2 tbsp white wine vinegar
- ¼ cup of finely sliced fresh dill
- One clove of garlic, minced
- ½ tsp sugar
- Freshly ground black Pepper, as needed

INSTRUCTIONS

After halving the cucumber, cut every half lengthwise down the middle. To remove the seeds from the middle, use the tsp tip. Slice every half thinly, then add the pieces of red onion to a sieve. Add some salt, then let it rest in the sink until the water runs out—at least 30 minutes.

In a medium-sized bowl, prepare the dressing by mixing the sour cream, mayonnaise, white wine vinegar, garlic, dill, sugar, and black Pepper.

When the onions and cucumbers are done, use a big wad of paper towels to pat the veggies dry after releasing any extra water by tapping the colander against the sink's base. Mix well after adding the dressing. Once ready to serve, cover and refrigerate.

Set the grill's temperature to medium-high. After cleaning, give the grill rack an oil brush. Shut the cover and let the temperature rise again. After rubbing the salmon with olive oil, liberally season it with kosher salt and Pepper. After placing the fillets skin side down, grill them for 4 to 5 minutes or until golden brown and slightly charred. Avoid peeking or flipping the fillets too soon since they should release quickly after beautifully searing them on the first side. Grill the fillets for two to three minutes or until they are done. Let it cool, peel it if desired, and serve with the chilled cucumber-dill salad on top or as a side dish.

NUTRITION INFORMATION
Per serving (4 servings)

522 calories, Fat: 39g, 9g of it saturated, 6g of carbohydrates, 3g of sugar, 1g of fiber, 36g of protein, 706mg of sodium, and 108mg of cholesterol.

28. CHICKEN CASSEROLE RECIPE

Prep Time: 10 minutes

Cook Time: 6 hours 20 minutes

Total Time: 6 hours 30 minutes

Servings: 4

Ingredients

- 2 tbsp vegetable oil
- 8 boneless chicken thighs trimmed of fat
- 2 tbsp unsalted butter
- 2 brown onions peeled and diced
- 3 cloves garlic peeled and minced
- 3 tbsp plain (all-purpose) flour
- 1 tsp salt
- 1 tsp black Pepper
- 1 tsp dried thyme
- ½ tsp celery salt
- 480 ml (2 cup ofs) chicken stock
- 1 tbsp freshly squeezed lemon juice

- 16-20 baby chestnut mushrooms
- 16-20 chantenay carrots
- 3 sticks of celery roughly chopped
- 60 ml (1/4 cup of) double (heavy) cream
- small bunch of parsley chopped

Instructions

Grease a large frying pan with oil over medium-high heat.
Twist-up of vegetable oil
It should take around five minutes to add the chicken thighs and gently brown them on both sides.
Eight deboned chicken thighs
After browning, remove them from the pan and put them in the slow cooker.
Melt the butter after adding it to the pan.
One tbsp of unsalted butter
Add the onion and simmer, turning occasionally, until softened, about 5 minutes.
Two caramelized onions
Stir in the garlic and heat for a Another minute.
Three garlic cloves
Add the flour, celery salt, thyme, Pepper, and salt and stir. Simmer for two minutes.
Three tbsp plain (all-purpose) flour, one tsp of salt, black Pepper, dried thyme, and half a tsp of celery salt
Pour in the lemon juice and stock. Spoon mixture over chicken in slow cooker after stirring and heating to a boil.
Two cups of (480 ml) of chicken stock, one tbsp of freshly squeezed lemon juice
Stir the celery, carrots, and mushrooms into the slow cooker.
16–20 baby carrots, 16–20 chantey mushrooms, and 3 stalks of celery

After covering, cook for five to six hours on low or three to four hours on high heat.

60 ml (1/4 cup of) thick double cream
Serve with fresh parsley on top. This dish is so delicious and served with green beans and mashed potatoes.
It's a little bunch of parsley.

Nutrition

Calories: 422kcal | Carbohydrates: 19g | Protein: 32g | Fat: 25g | Cholesterol: 172mg | Sodium: 1597mg | Potassium: 984mg | Fiber: 3g | Sugar: 7g | Vitamin A: 6081IU | Vitamin C: 8mg | Calcium: 87mg | Iron: 3mg .

29. EASY BAKED CHICKEN

PREP TIME 5MINUTES

COOK TIME 25MINUTES

TOTAL TIME 30MINUTES

SERVINGS 6

INGREDIENTS

- 5-6 Boneless Skinless Chicken Breasts
- 2 Tbsp Olive Oil
- 1/2 tsp Paprika
- 1 tsp Italian Seasoning
- 1 tsp Salt
- 1 tsp Pepper

INSTRUCTIONS

Heat the oven to 400°F before baking.

The chicken breast should be put in a 9 x 13 baking dish.

Coat chicken breasts lightly with olive oil. I coated the chicken breasts with a basting brush.

In a small dish, mix all the spices.

Cover chicken breasts with a spice mixture.

The chicken should reach 165 degrees Fahrenheit inside after 25 to 30 minutes of uncovered baking.

Before slicing, let every chicken breast rest for at least five minutes.

Have fun!

NUTRITION FACTS

Calories 151kcal, Carbohydrates 1g, Protein 20g, Fat 7g, Cholesterol 60mg, Sodium 497mg, Potassium 348mg, Fiber 1g, Sugar 1g, Calcium 10mg, Iron 1mg.

30. BASIL PESTO CHICKEN PASTA

PREP TIME 5minutes

COOK TIME 15minutes

TOTAL TIME 20minutes

SERVINGS 2 people

INGREDIENTS

- 8 Ounces chicken breast skinless, boneless (230g)
- 2 tbsp extra virgin olive oil
- Himalayan salt as needed
- Black Pepper as need
- 1 cup of green beans
- 1 ½ cup of whole wheat penne pasta
- Parmesan cheese Parmigiano-Reggiano or Grana Padano, freshly grated
- For Basil Pesto
- 2 cups of fresh basil
- 4 tbsp walnuts
- ½ cup of Parmesan cheese Parmigiano-Reggiano or Grana Padano, freshly grated
- ½ avocado OR ½ cup of extra virgin olive oil
- 1 tsp lemon juice
- Himalayan salt as needed

INSTRUCTIONS

Heat the olive oil in the deeper, bigger pan over medium heat. Add the smaller-cut chicken pieces. Once browned on both sides, fry the chicken for 8 to 10 minutes. As needed, add more salt and Pepper. Take the pan off of the burner.

Meanwhile, give the green beans a 10-minute boil before draining. Before the pasta is al dente, cook it in salted water as directed on the package. Save the pasta water after draining the noodles.

Toss the cooked pasta and beans into the pan with the chicken. Mix well after adding 3 tbsp of basil pesto. If the pasta seems too dry, add one or two tsp of water to boil it.

Present warm, garnished with freshly grated Parmesan cheese.

Regarding Basil Pesto

Add the walnuts and fresh basil to a food processor and mince.

Grated cheese and, if used, garlic should be added and mixed with another. Scrape the mixture from the bowl walls with a rubber spatula.

Add the avocado and stir until the mixture is smooth. If the mixture is too thick, add some olive oil. Alternately, stir in olive oil instead of the avocado until a smooth pesto is achieved.

Place the pesto into a jar and seal it shut. Refrigerate for a maximum of two weeks.x

NUTRITION

Calories: 518kcal | Carbohydrates: 40g | Protein: 33g | Fat: 29g | Cholesterol: 72mg | Sodium: 448mg | Potassium: 335mg | Fiber: 8g | Sugar: 4g | Vitamin A: 1600IU | Vitamin C: 30.5mg | Calcium: 190mg | Iron: 3.1mg .

31. GROUND CHICKEN SHEPHERD'S PIE

PREP TIME 5minutes

COOK TIME 30minutes

TOTAL TIME 35minutes

SERVINGS 4

INGREDIENTS

- For the base of the Shepherd's Pie:
- 1 lb minced chicken
- ½ cup of carrots peeled, cubed
- ½ cup of peas
- ½ cup of French beans
- 1 red onion chopped

- 2 tomato pureed
- 3 cloves garlic
- 2 tbsp olive oil extra virgin
- 1 tbsp almond flour
- 1 tsp Worcestershire sauce
- 3 sprigs thyme
- 2 bay leaf dried
- 1 cinnamon
- ½ tsp cayenne powder
- 1½ tsp salt
- 1 tsp pepper powder
- 3 sprigs parsley for garnish
- For the mashed potatoes:
- 2 Russet potato
- 2 tbsp unsalted butter
- 1 tbsp whole milk
- a pinch salt
- ⅛ tsp pepper

INSTRUCTIONS
How to make the base:
Smoothly blend the tomatoes and garlic, then leave aside.

Add the cinnamon, thyme, bay leaf, and olive oil to a heated Dutch oven.

For two minutes, add the onion and sauté. After that, sauté the tomato-garlic puree for three minutes.

Remove the entire spices and the thyme. Cook for four minutes after adding the seasonings and ground chicken.

Stir in the vegetables and ¼ cup of water to thaw. Cook for five minutes until evaporated but the consistency is still somewhat wet.

Method for mashing potatoes:
Add pressure. For fifteen minutes, simmer or boil the potatoes. After peeling the skin, mash them with a masher. Beat in the salt and Pepper using a fork.

Warm up a skillet, add the milk, butter, and mashed potatoes, and stir for one or two minutes. Let the mixture cool.

The Ground Chicken Shepherd's Pie assembly instructions:
Smooth the ground chicken-veggie mixture on top of the bottom of an oval 9-inch pie plate.

Place dollops of the base mixture onto the mashed potato mixture.

Using your fork, smooth out the top and Make a crisscross pattern. Make sure to tightly seal the borders to prevent the base mixture from expanding.

Bake until the tops are golden brown, about 10 minutes at 4000F and 5 minutes at 4250F.

Take a piece and serve it with parsley-topped sour cream.

NUTRITION

Calories: 348kcal, Carbohydrates: 32g, Protein: 25g, Fat: 18g, Cholesterol: 98mg, Sodium: 980mg, Potassium: 1397mg, Fiber: 5g , Sugar: 6g , Vitamin A: 3741IU , Vitamin C: 30mg , Calcium: 77mg, Iron: 3mg.

32. STEAK-AND-POTATO SALAD

Total: 35 min

Active: 35 min

Yield: 4 servings

Ingredients

- 1 1/4 pounds quartered little red potatoes
- For brushing, add
- extra virgin olive oil (approximately 1/4 cup).
- kosher salt with just-ground Pepper
- 3 tbsp steak sauce
- One tbsp of vinegar made from red wine
- 2 tsp Dijon mustard
- 1 1/2 pounds of boneless, 1-inch-thick sirloin steak
- 2 ripped romaine lettuce hearts
- 1 large beefsteak tomato, quartered and sliced
- 1/4 cup of fresh chives, chopped; add more for garnish
- 1/2 cup of crumbled blue cheese

Directions

Put racks in the oven's top and bottom positions. On the bottom rack, set a baking sheet with a rim. Start the oven at 450 degrees Fahrenheit. Toss potatoes in a bowl with two tbsp of olive oil, half a tsp of salt, and a few grinds of Pepper. Spread onto the heated pan and bake for 18 to 20 minutes, rotating once or until golden and tender.

In the meantime, mix the remaining 2 tbsp of olive oil, vinegar, mustard, and steak sauce in a big bowl; leave aside. Over high heat, heat a large ovenproof skillet. Dredge the steak in olive oil on both sides, then season with salt and Pepper. Add to the skillet and cook for approximately 2 minutes on every side or until browned. Use roughly 1 tbsp of the vinaigrette to coat the steak's top lightly. After moving the pan to the top oven rack, cook the steak for about 4 minutes, or until a thermometer inserted sideways into it reads 120 degrees F for medium-rare. After moving it to a chopping board and giving it a five-minute rest, thinly cut it against the grain.

Incorporate two tbsp of the skillet's juices into the vinaigrette bowl. Toss in the romaine lettuce, tomato, and chives after seasoning with salt and Pepper. After dividing the salad among plates, add the steak, potatoes, blue cheese, and more chives.

CHAPTER FOUR: BREAKFAST

33. PEAR, BANANA, OAT AND HONEY BREAKFAST SMOOTHIE RECIPE

5 minutes to prepare

250 calories/serving

Serves 2

Ingredients

- 1 ripe, juicy pear, cored
- 1 ripe banana, peeled
- 30g porridge oats
- 1 tbsp clear honey
- 110g low-fat natural yogurt

- 250ml apple juice
- handful ice cubes

Method

In a food processor or smoothie maker, mix all the ingredients and process until smooth.
Chill and pour into a large glass.

Every serving contains

Energy1075kj, 250kcal13, Fat2g3, Saturates1g5, Sugars 48g53, Salt 0.5g<1 .

34. SUMMER BERRY PARFAIT WITH YOGURT AND GRANOLA

Prep Time:10 mins

Total Time:10 mins

Servings:1

Yield:1 serving

Ingredients

- ¾ cup of sliced strawberries
- ¾ cup of blueberries
- 1 (6-ounce) container of vanilla yogurt
- 1 tbsp wheat germ
- ½ banana, sliced
- ⅓ cup of granola

Directions

Arrange 1/4 cup of blueberries, 1/4 cup of strawberries, 1/3 container yogurt, 1/3 tbsp wheat germ, 1/3 of the banana slices, and around 2 tbsp of granola onto a large platter. Once every ingredient has been utilized, layer the parfait and build it up.

Nutrition Facts (per serving)

521	Calories
14g	Fat
87g	Carbs
18g	Protein

35. PROTEIN PORRIDGE

Prep:5 mins

Cook:5 mins

Serves 1

Ingredients

- 40g oats (use gluten-free, if needed)
- 250ml liquid (milk, nut milk, or half milk/half water will work), + an extra 1-2 tbsp
- 15g protein powder
- 1 tsp ground cinnamon
- 1 tsp vanilla extract

Toppings (optional):

- granola
- banana slices
- chocolate chips
- shelled hemp seeds

Method

To make the oats thick and creamy, add the liquid and oats to a pan and simmer over medium heat for two to three minutes. Reduce the heat and blend in the protein powder until well-mixed. Add a couple more sips of liquid vanilla and cinnamon, and whisk for an additional minute until the mixture becomes lusciously creamy. Please turn off the heat slightly before the mixture achieves the ideal texture since it will thicken as it cools.

Transfer the porridge onto a bowl and present it with the garnishing components. Hemp seeds are a fantastic option for an extra protein boost.

36. SPINACH FETA OMELET

PREP TIME: 5minutes

COOK TIME: 5minutes

TOTAL TIME: 10minutes

SERVINGS: 1 Person

Ingredients

- 1 tsp olive oil

- 1 cup of baby spinach
- As needed, add freshly ground Pepper and Kosher salt.
- 2 to 3 large eggs
- 1 tbsp of butter without salt
- ¼ cup of crumbled feta (or goat cheese)
- Two tsp finely chopped fresh chives for decoration (optional)

Instructions

Over medium-high heat, heat an 8-inch omelet pan or shallow skillet (ideally nonstick). After heating the olive oil, add the spinach, sprinkle with salt and Pepper, and toss for one minute or until the spinach wilts. Move to a little plate.

Once the eggs are cracked into a small bowl, beat them with a fork to include the salt and Pepper.

Put the pan back on the burner and stir in the butter. Once it has melted, swirl the pan to ensure that the bottom is equally coated. Once the eggs are added to the pan, rapidly shake and swirl the pan to ensure the eggs coat the whole bottom. After the eggs have been set on the bottom, which should take around 30 seconds, raise the omelet's edges with a rubber spatula so that any raw egg on top may slide below. Add the feta and sautéed spinach to half the eggs, then heat for 30 seconds. The top should be somewhat wet but not overly runny (unless that's how you prefer it). Place the untopped side of the eggs onto a platter and flip it over the filling. If desired, garnish with fresh chives.

Nutrition

368KCAL, 3G of carbohydrates, 17G of protein, 32G of fat, 391MG of cholesterol, 569MG of sodium, 321MG of potassium, 1G of fiber, 2G of sugar, 3883IU of vitamin A, 10MG of vitamin C, 269MG of calcium, and 3MG of iron.

37. SPINACH PARMESAN BAKED EGGS RECIPE

Serving Size 1 egg with 1/2 cup of spinach mixture

Ingredients

- 2 tsp olive oil
- 2 garlic cloves minced
- 4 cup of baby spinach
- 1/2 cup of parmesan cheese fat-free, grated
- 4 eggs
- 1 tomato small, diced small

Instructions

Set the oven's temperature to 350. Add nonstick spray to an 8 x 8-inch casserole dish.

In a large pan, preheat the olive oil over medium heat. Add the garlic and spinach once warm. Sauté the spinach until it begins to wilt. Take off the heat source and remove any leftover liquid. After adding the parmesan cheese, uniformly put the mixture into the casserole dish.

Make four little indentations in the spinach to hold the eggs. Place one egg into every crevice. Bake until the egg whites are almost set, 15 to 20 minutes. Take it out of the oven, allow it to cool for approximately five minutes, and then top with the tomato. Present and savor!

Nutrition Information

There are 149 calories, 12 grams of protein, 3 grams of carbs, 170 mg of cholesterol, 10 grams of fat, 280 mg of sodium, and 1 gram of sugar.

38. SALMON AND EGGS

PREP TIME: 5 MINUTES

COOK TIME: 5 MINUTES

TOTAL TIME: 10 MINUTES

SERVINGS: 2

Ingredients
FOR THE EGGS AND SALMON

- 4 large eggs
- 2 tbsp half and half*
- 1/8 tsp salt
- 1 tbsp ghee or butter
- Four ounces of chunky hot-roasted smoked salmon**
- 1/4 cup of freshly cut fresh chives
- freshly ground black Pepper

COMPATIBLE PAIRINGS

- fresh avocado slices
- hash browns
- drop biscuits

Instructions

Set the oven's temperature to 350. Add nonstick spray to an 8 x 8-inch casserole dish.

In a large saucepan set over medium heat, warm the olive oil. Add the garlic and spinach once heated. Sauté the spinach until it begins to wilt. Take off the heat source and remove any leftover liquid. After adding the parmesan cheese, uniformly put the mixture into the casserole dish.

Make four little indentations in the spinach to hold the eggs. Place one egg into every crevice. Bake until the egg whites are almost set, 15 to 20 minutes. Take it out of the oven, allow it to cool for approximately five minutes, and then top with the tomato. Present and savor!

Nutrition

calories: 243 kcal, 1g of carbs, 24g of protein, 15g of fat, 409 mg of cholesterol, 318 mg of sodium, 435 mg of potassium, 1g of sugar, 616 IU of vitamin A, 1 mg of vitamin C, 79 mg of calcium, and 2 mg of iron

39. RICOTTA AND SPINACH FRITTATA WITH MINT

Total Time: 30 minutes

Yield: Six servings

INGREDIENTS

- 6ounces fresh spinach stemmed and washed, or ½ 6-ounce bag baby spinach
- 6eggs
- Salt
- freshly ground Pepper
- 1cup of fresh ricotta
- 1tbsp chopped fresh mint
- 1garlic clove, minced
- 2tbsp olive oil

PREPARATION

For around two minutes, or until the spinach wilts, place it over an inch of boiling water to steam. Squeeze off extra moisture, rinse with cold water, and finely chop.

Beat the eggs, ricotta, garlic, spinach, mint, salt, and pepper in a medium-sized bowl.

Lightly heat the olive oil in a heavy-duty 10-inch nonstick pan over medium-high heat. If a small egg amount is dropped into the pan and immediately sizzles and cooks, the pan is ready. Transfer the egg mixture in. To uniformly spread the eggs and stuffing throughout the surface, tilt the pan. To allow the eggs to flow beneath during the first few minutes of cooking, gently shake the pan and tilt it slightly with one hand while pushing up the frittata's borders with the spatula in your other hand.

Turn down the heat to low, cover, and cook for ten minutes, impartially shaking the pan. Tilt the pan, remove the cover periodically, and loosen the bottom with a wooden spatula to avoid the frittata's bottom from burning. It should grow golden in hue. If the eggs aren't almost set, cook them for a few more minutes.

As you wait, heat the broiler. Remove the pan's lid and set it under the broiler, keeping it slightly off the heat source for one to three minutes. Watch closely to ensure the top doesn't burn; at most, it should puff and brown slightly under the broiler. Take the frittata off the heat and let it cool for at least five minutes and up to fifteen minutes, shaking the pan to ensure it doesn't cling. Loosen the edges of the pan with a wooden or plastic spatula, then carefully transfer it to a large circular dish. It is sliced into smaller diamonds, around the size of a mouthful. Serve warm, room temperature, chilly, or hot.

40. HEARTY BREAKFAST BURRITOS

Prep Time 20 minutes

Cook Time 30 minutes

Total Time 50 minutes

8 Burritos

Ingredients

- 1 cup of jasmine rice
- 1 1/2 cups of water

- 2 bell peppers
- 1 tsp oil
- 1 pound breakfast sausage
- 1 dozen eggs
- 1 cup of milk
- 2 tsp salt
- 1 tbsp butter
- 2 cups of cheddar cheese grated
- 8 tsp hot sauce
- 8 tbsp ranch dressing
- 8 10-inch flour tortillas

Instructions

In a heavy-bottomed saucepan, mix the rice and water. Bring a boil, then simmer for eighteen minutes on low heat with a lid on. Once the heat is off, let the rice rest for 10 minutes. Using a fork, fluff.

Cut the bell peppers lengthwise. The peppers should be cooked for 8 to 10 minutes over medium heat in a skillet with oil added, then left aside.

Sausage should be browned in a skillet over medium heat before being put aside.

Whisk together the eggs, milk, and salt. Set a pan over medium heat and melt the butter. When the eggs are done, add them, cook, and set aside.

Place 1/8 of the rice, peppers, sausage, eggs, and cheese in the middle of every tortilla once it has been laid out. Add one tsp of spicy sauce and one tbsp of ranch dressing. Fold the left and right sides together, leaving approximately an inch of space between the left and right edges. Roll into a burrito by folding the bottom toward the top. Continue making the final seven burritos.

Wrap aluminum foil around every tortilla.

Nutrition

Calories: 625kcal | Carbohydrates: 38g | Protein: 29g | Fat: 38g | Cholesterol: 324mg | Sodium: 1626mg | Potassium: 441mg | Fiber: 1g | Sugar: 4g | Vitamin A: 1715IU | Vitamin C: 42.1mg | Calcium: 324mg | Iron: 3.3mg .

41. TURKEY HASH BROWN BREAKFAST CASSEROLE

Servings: 8

Ingredients

- 1 lb lean ground turkey
- 1 tbsp oil
- 1 small onion chopped
- 12 large eggs lightly beaten
- 1 tsp salt
- 1/2 tsp pepper
- 1 tsp Italian Herbs
- One container of sixteen ounces of thawed frozen shredded hash brown potatoes
- 1 cup of 4 ounces 2% shredded cheddar cheese

Instructions

Add the chopped onion in a massive pan with hot oil and sauté it for a few minutes.

Next, add the ground turkey, sprinkle with the Italian herbs, and cook, turning regularly, over medium-high heat for three to four minutes.

In a bowl, beat the eggs with the salt and Pepper.

Add the turkey, onions, half of the cheese, and hash browns to the bowl with the eggs.

Transfer to a 13 x9-inch baking dish that has been greased, and then sprinkle the remaining cheese on top.

Bake for 35 to 45 minutes, uncovered, at 350°, or until a knife inserted near the middle comes out clean.

CHAPTER FIVE: VEGETARIAN

42. TAHINI BANANA DATE SHAKES

Total Time: 5 minutes

Yield: 3 cups of

INGREDIENTS

- 2 frozen bananas, sliced
- 4 pitted Medjool dates (if they're too big, you can chop them up a bit.)
- ¼ cup of tahini (I used Soom tahini)
- ¼ cup of crushed ice
- 1 ½ cups of unsweetened almond milk
- Pinch ground cinnamon, more for later

INSTRUCTIONS

After slicing the frozen bananas, add the remaining ingredients to your blender. Blend until a creamy, smooth shake is produced. Spoon the banana-date shakes into serving glasses and garnish with a little more of the ground cinnamon. Have fun!

43. KEFIR GREEN SMOOTHIE

yield: 1-2 SERVINGS

prep time: 5 MINUTES

total time: 5 MINUTES

YIELD: 1 SERVING SIZE: 1

INGREDIENTS

- 1 ½ cup ofs milk kefir
- 2 cups of loosely packed baby spinach
- 1 cup of fresh (frozen mango chunks)
- 1 cup of fresh (frozen pineapple chunks)
- 1 medium banana, peeled
- 1 tbsp maple syrup (optional)

INSTRUCTIONS

Transfer your milk kefir and spinach into a premium blender jar.

Blend the spinach with the milk kefir by processing it well at a high speed.

Stir in the banana and frozen fruit. If using maple syrup, you can add it now.

Blend on high until extremely smooth.

Transfer into a glass jar or tumbler and decorate with a large straw.

Be present and relish!

NUTRITION INFORMATION:

Amount per serving: Calories: 597, total fat: 5g, trans fat: 0g, unsaturated fat: 2g, Cholesterol: 16mg, Sodium: 763mg, carbohydrates: 126g, fiber: 10gsugar: 107g, protein: 22g.

44. CHICKPEA SALAD

Prep Time: 20 minutes

Total Time: 20 minutes

Serves 4 to 6

Ingredients

- Two tsp of pure olive oil
- two tsp freshly squeezed lemon juice
- one clove of grated garlic
- 1 tsp Dijon mustard
- 1 tsp sea salt
- Three cups of cooked, rinsed, and drained chickpeas
- Two cups of half-cut mixed red and yellow grape tomatoes

- ½ Diced
- English cucumber
- ½ cup of pickled red onions
- ½ cup of pitted and halved Kalamata olives
- ½ cup of freshly chopped parsley
- ¼ cup of freshly chopped dill
- Add ¼ cup of finely chopped fresh mint leaves as a garnish.
- Recently ground black Pepper.

Instructions

Mix the olive oil, lemon juice, mustard, garlic, salt, and a few Pepper grinds in a big bowl.

Toss to coat the chickpeas, tomatoes, cucumber, olives, and pickled onions. Toss one more after adding the mint, dill, and parsley.

Serve as a garnish with fresh mint leaves and season to suit.

45. CAPRESE SALAD RECIPE

Prep Time: 10 minutes

Refrigerate: 15minutes

Total Time: 25minutes

Ingredients

- 1-pint cherry tomatoes, sliced in half
- 2 Tbsp olive oil
- 2 Tbsp balsamic vinegar
- ½ tsp salt

- ¼ tsp pepper
- ¼ tsp dried oregano or thyme
- ¼ cup of chopped basil
- 1 cup of mozzarella balls
- Balsamic glaze for serving

Instructions

Mix the tomatoes, mozzarella balls and

I just chopped basil in a big dish.

Balsamic vinegar, olive oil, salt, Pepper, and dried oregano should all be combined in a small bowl.
Drizzle the tomato mixture with the dressing, then toss to blend. Keep chilled until you're ready to serve.
As needed, add additional salt, Pepper, or basil. If desired, drizzle with balsamic glaze.

Nutrition

102 kcal, 4g of carbohydrates, 4g of protein, 8g of fat, 6 mg of cholesterol, 216 mg of sodium, 178 mg of potassium, 1g of Fiber, 3g of sugar, 440 IU of vitamin A, 18.2 mg of vitamin C, 70 mg of calcium, and 0.6 mg of iron.

46. STUFFED JALAPENOS PEPPER RECIPE WITH RICOTTA CHEESE

Prep in 15 minutes

Cooks in 30 minutes

Total in 45 minutes

Makes: 4-5 Servings

Ingredients

- 10 Pickled Jalapenos or long red or green peppers (chilies)
- 100 grams Ricotta Cheese, or paneer, crumbled
- 1 Red Bell pepper (Capsicum), finely chopped
- Tabasco Original - Hot Sauce, as needed
- Salt and Pepper, as need
- 1/2 cup of Cheddar cheese, grated
- Oil, to cook

How to make Stuffed Jalapenos Pepper Recipe with Ricotta Cheese

To make the stuffed jalapeño pepper recipe with ricotta cheese, heat the oven to 200 degrees Celsius and coat a baking sheet with butter or oil. To make the stuffed jalapeño pepper recipe with ricotta cheese, heat the oven to 200 degrees Celsius and coat a baking sheet with butter or oil.

Add the red peppers and sauté over medium heat in a heavy-based pan with heated oil until they become tender and browned. Set aside.

Add the peppers, ricotta cheese, tabasco sauce, salt, and roughly ground black Pepper to a mixing bowl. Mix well by stirring.

After cutting the long Pepper or jalapeño in half lengthwise, scoop off the seeds and any leftover white skin membrane.

Spoon the cottage cheese mixture into every half of the jalapeños. Add a sprinkling of cheddar cheese.

Repeat with the remaining jalapeños and transfer to the baking sheet that has been oiled. Bake for five to ten minutes until the cheese is melted and the jalapeños' edges start to color.

Serve the Protein Fingers Recipe, the Fizzy Pomegranate & Mint Mocktail Recipe, and this Stuffed Jalapenos Pepper Recipe with Ricotta Cheese as a party starter.

47. PROTEIN BOWL (VEGAN BUDDHA BOWL)

PREP TIME:35MINUTES

COOK TIME:30MINUTES

TOTAL TIME:1HOUR 5MINUTES

SERVINGS: 4 BOWLS

Ingredients
Baked tofu

- One block Firm Tofu - drained
- 1 tbsp Sesame Oil
- 1 tbsp Cornstarch
- ¼ tsp Garlic Powder

- ¼ tsp Ground Ginger

For the 4 bowls

- 3 cups of Cooked Quinoa - equivalent 1 cup of uncooked
- ½ cup of Cabbage - thinly shredded
- ½ cup of Red Bell Pepper - thinly sliced
- 1 cup of Cooked Edamame - lukewarm
- 1 large Carrot - peeled, thinly sliced

Protein dressing

- ¼ cup of Almond Butter
- 3 tbsp Rice Vinegar
- 2 tsp Maple Syrup
- 2 tbsp Soy Sauce
- 1 tsp Sesame Oil
- ¼ tsp Garlic Powder
- ¼ tsp Red Chili Flakes
- 2-3 tbsp Coconut Milk
- 2 tsp Maple Syrup

Protein Toppings

- 2 tsp Hemp Seeds
- 1 tsp Sesame Seeds

Instructions

Heat the oven to 180°C, or 350°F. Add grease to the parchment paper. Line a baking sheet. Put aside.

To help you, prepare 1 cup of Quinoa according to the directions on the package or use my rice cooker quinoa lesson.

The tofu should be wrapped in absorbent kitchen paper, put on a dish, and then covered with a heavy object, such as a cookbook. Hold off for ten minutes.

Meanwhile, whisk together the Cornstarch, ginger, garlic powder, and sesame oil to make the tofu marinade in a mixing dish.

Sliced and drained tofu should be placed in a bowl with the marinade and stirred to coat. Allocate ten minutes.

Without touching them, arrange the tofu cubes on the baking sheet. Bake, rotating them halfway through, for 25 to 30 minutes or until golden and crispy.

Meanwhile, finely cut the carrots, Cabbage, and red bell pepper. Put aside.

Cook the Edamame according to the package's directions. I pour boiling water over frozen Edamame, then drain and use lukewarm in the recipe. Put aside.

All the almond butter dressing ingredients should be mixed in a nonstick saucepan, heated to medium, and gently whisk until thickened.

Add the cubes of baked tofu to the heavy sauce and stir.

Add an equal quantity of tofu (100g every) and raw veggies to the bottom of every bowl after dividing the cooked Quinoa (3/4 cup of every) to construct the bowls.

For an added protein and crunch boost, sprinkle some seeds on top.

Storage

Keep leftovers in a sealed container for up to three days in the refrigerator.

Consume warm or cold.

Nutrition

Serving: 1bowl | Calories: 495.5kcal | Carbohydrates: 48.3g | Protein: 24.8g | Fat: 23.8g |
Sodium: 525.7mg | Potassium: 625.2mg | Fiber: 9.3g | Sugar: 8.7g

| Vitamin A: 661.6IU | Vitamin B12: 0.1µg | Vitamin C: 29.4mg | Vitamin D: 3.8µg | Calcium: 253.3mg | Iron: 5.5mg | Magnesium: 169.5mg | Phosphorus: 408.8mg | Zinc: 2.8mg .

48. SPICY MANGO, BLACK BEAN & AVOCADO TACOS

Serves: 2

Ingredients

- 4 to 6 tortillas, lightly charred or warmed (I like La Tortilla Factory White Corn or homemade tortillas)
- 1 cup of cooked, rinsed, and drained black beans
- 2 limes divided
- ¼ to ½ tsp chili powder*
- 2 cups of shredded green Cabbage
- ½ avocado, thinly sliced
- ½ mango, diced
- 2 tbsp chopped cilantro
- 2 tbsp crumbled feta or cotija cheese
- sliced serrano pepper and additional sriracha for serving, optional*
- sea salt

Instructions

Mix the black beans, one tbsp lime juice, ¼ to ½ tsp chile powder, and ¼ tsp salt in a small dish.

Prepare the hot mayonnaise: Mix the sriracha and mayonnaise in a small bowl.

Give the Cabbage a couple of pinches of salt and a tsp of lime juice.

Spoon the Cabbage, avocado slices, black beans, mango, cilantro, spicy mayo, and feta cheese into every tortilla. Serve the tacos with more sriracha and sliced serrano peppers for a hotter version. Slices of lime are served alongside.

49. HUMMUS QUESADILLAS!

Prep Time: 7 mins

Cook Time: 8 mins

Total Time: 15 minutes

Yield: 1

INGREDIENTS
Per quesadilla

- One 8-inch whole-grain tortilla (or one without gluten for quesadillas without gluten)
- ¼ to ⅓ cup of hummus of choice (green goddess hummus is my favorite)
- One 8-inch whole-grain tortilla (or one without gluten for quesadillas without gluten)
- Extra-virgin olive oil for brushing
- Optional for serving: additional hummus, hot sauce, pesto, etc.

INSTRUCTIONS

Drizzle a thick layer of hummus onto your tortilla. Gently stuff one half of the tortilla with your preferred contents. To form a half-moon, fold the blank side over. You may cook up to two quesadillas at a time in the same skillet if you'd like to make more.

Heat a skillet to a medium temperature. Fold the quesadilla(s) and place them in the pan. After a minute or two, let the bottom sides warm up before carefully flipping. Give the heated sides a quick coat of olive oil and allow them to continue cooking for a minute or two more. Once again, carefully turn, gently spray the new top side with olive oil, and cook until the bottom is crisp and faintly brown. Cook, flipping carefully, until the other side is crisp and faintly brown.

After moving the quesadilla(s) to a chopping board, let them rest for a few minutes. Then, cut every quesadilla into three wedges using a sharp chef's knife or pie cutter. Serve right away. I ate mine just how I liked it, but you might try adding more hummus, spicy sauce, or pesto on the side.

CHAPTER SIX: SEAFOOD

50. NO-MAYO MEDITERRANEAN TUNA

Prep Time: 5 mins

Additional Time: 30 mins

Total Time: 35 mins

Servings: 2

Yield: 2 servings

Ingredients

- 1 6-ounces can of drained tuna in water
- 3 tbsp mayonnaise
- 2 tbsp hummus spread
- 8 olives, chopped or more as needed
- 1 tsp dried oregano, or more according to preference
- salt and ground black Pepper as needed

Directions

Flake the tuna into a small container using a fork. Add the olives, hummus, and mayonnaise. Add the Pepper, salt, and oregano. After thoroughly combining all the ingredients, chill them for around half an hour.

51. TUNA WRAPS

Prep Time: 10 minutes

Total Time: 10 minutes

Servings: 2 wraps

Ingredients

- Five-ounce can of drained, water-packed tuna
- ¼ cup of mayo (no sugar added)
- 2 tbsp of finely chopped onions of your preferred variety
- ½ cup of finely sliced lettuce (I used romaine)
- ¼ tsp of salt
- 2 standard whole-grain tortillas

Instructions

Mix the tuna, mayo, onions, and salt in a dish.
With a fork, thoroughly blend.
Arrange your tortilla or wrapper.
Line a baking sheet with lettuce, then top with half the tuna salad.
Tightly roll the wrap as much as you can.
Divide in two.
Assist.

Nutrition

Serving: 1wrap | Calories: 291kcal | Carbohydrates: 2g | Protein: 17g | Fat: 23g | Cholesterol: 42mg | Sodium: 744mg | Potassium: 214mg | Fiber: 1g | Sugar: 1g | Calcium: 20mg | Iron: 1mg

52. SHRIMP POKE BOWL RECIPE [SWEET SOY GLAZE + SPICY MAYONNAISE]

Total Time: 1 hour 40 minutes

Yield: 4 servings

INGREDIENTS
MARINATED SHRIMP & SWEET SOY GLAZE:

- 40–50 medium shrimp (fresh or frozen), peeled and deveined
- 1/4 cup of soy sauce
- 2 tbsp honey
- 1 tbsp rice vinegar
- 1 tsp sesame oil
- 1 tsp sriracha

GINGER TURMERIC COCONUT RICE:

- This coconut rice recipe
- 1 small (2-3 inch) piece fresh ginger
- 1 small (2-3 inch) piece of fresh turmeric
- approximately 1/4 cup of water

PICKLED CARROTS:

- 3 large carrots, peeled into long strips
- 1 cup of water
- 1/2 cup of white vinegar
- 1/2 cup of rice vinegar (genuine brewed)
- 1/4 cup of pure cane sugar

- 1 tbsp pickling or kosher salt
- 1 tsp fresh garlic, minced

SPICY MAYONNAISE:

- 1/2 cup of mayonnaise
- 3 tbsp sriracha (less if you're sensitive to heat)
- 2 tsp lime juice
- 1/2 tsp water
- 1/8 tsp sesame oil

TOPPINGS:

- 1 avocado, sliced
- 1/2 cup of shelled Edamame (fresh or frozen)
- 1/2 cup of mango or pineapple (fresh or frozen), diced
- 1/4 cup of scallions, sliced
- several sheets of nori/seaweed snacks cut into strips
- a handful of microgreens
- 3 tbsp sesame seeds, toasted (see instructions below)
- One lime, cut into wedges

INSTRUCTIONS

Pat your (defrosted, peeled, and deveined) shrimp dry before marinating them. See the notes below if your honey has crystallized or is challenging to handle. Mix the soy sauce, honey, rice vinegar, sesame oil, and sriracha in a medium-sized bowl. While preparing the other ingredients, toss the shrimp in the marinade, cover it, and place it in the refrigerator.

Rice: You may start with regular rice, but I highly recommend this ginger turmeric coconut rice recipe. Start by following the directions for the Fluffy Coconut Rice recipe. *NOTE: Make sure you have time for this since it takes an hour to soak the rice thoroughly. If you want to add ginger or turmeric juice to the cooked coconut rice, mix some ginger and turmeric with water, then filter using a rubber spatula or fine-mesh strainer. Either pour all the juice over the cooked rice or offer it as an alternative to be served separately.

Easy Pickled Carrots: *For pre-pickling instructions, see the notes below! Put the rice and white vinegar, sugar, salt, and water in a small saucepan. To dissolve the sugar, cover and bring the mixture to a boil. With a vegetable peeler, peel and slice the carrots into thin strips. Put them and the minced garlic in a mason jar. Drizzle the carrots with the hot pickling liquid, cover, and place in the fridge. If you're pressed for time, you can decide not to pickle the carrots.

Spicy Mayonnaise: Process mayonnaise, sriracha, lime juice, water, and sesame oil in a food processor. Process until well mixed and smooth. Could you put it in the fridge to chill?

Prepare the shrimp and sweet soy glaze by straining the marinade and transferring the shrimp to a small saucepan. To prevent burning, boil the marinade for at least five minutes while stirring. Set aside as it begins to thicken somewhat to solidify into a glaze. Put a skillet, such as a cast iron, over medium-high heat. Once the shrimp reach 145 degrees Fahrenheit (63 degrees Celsius), sauté them on every side for one to two minutes. The shrimp will become firm to the touch and turn pink in color.

Assemble after preparing the toppings: In a small pan over medium-high heat, toast or warm the sesame seeds, being careful to flip them frequently so they toast rather than burn. As listed in the ingredients list above, chop or dice the remaining components. Spoon a generous portion of rice into every bowl, then around the bowl with the toppings. Top with sesame seeds and a squeeze of lime juice, then drizzle with spicy mayonnaise and sweet soy glaze. Enjoy your shrimp poke bowls now!

53. GARLIC SHRIMP WITH QUINOA

PREP:5 minutes

COOK:25 minutes

TOTAL:30 minutes

SERVINGS: 4 servings

Ingredients

- 4 tsp of split pure virgin olive oil
- 1 pound raw, peeled, deveined shrimp (26–30counts) with tails
- 1 tsp divided of kosher salt
- 1/2 tsp chili powder divided
- About half of one small onion or 1/3 cup of finely chopped yellow onion
- 3 minced garlic cloves (approximately one tbsp)
- 1 cup of uncooked Quinoa
- 1/4 tsp cayenne pepper
- 1 cup of chicken broth

reduced in sodium

- 1 huge lemon
- Three tbsp fresh parsley, extra for garnish

Instructions

Heat 2 tsp olive oil in a big, tight-fitting nonstick pan over medium-high heat.

After adding the shrimp, mix with 1/4 tsp chile powder and 1/2 tsp salt. For approximately three minutes, or until the shrimp are pink and cooked through, sauté them. To avoid overcooking, take the shrimp right away and transfer them to a platter.

Warm the last two tablespoons of olive oil in the same pan as the onion. Allow to simmer for about 5 minutes or until the onion softens. Add the garlic and heat for approximately 30 seconds or until fragrant.

Add the cayenne, the remaining 1/2 tsp salt, and 1/4 tsp chile powder and stir. Allow the Quinoa to brown for two minutes after stirring to coat it with oil.

After adding the chicken stock, turn the heat high and boil the liquid. After it boils, turn down the heat to a simmer and cover. Simmer for 12 to 15 minutes or until the Quinoa is cooked. Take a fork and uncover and fluff.

First, zest the lemon and squeeze its juice into the pan. Next, add the lemon juice and parsley to the skillet. Add the reserved shrimp on top after tossing to mix. Add a little more fresh parsley on top. Warm up and serve.

Nutrition

Serving: 1(of 4)calories: 343kcal, carbohydrates: 34g, fat: 9g, protein: 32g, cholesterol: 286mg, potassium: 514mg, Fiber: 4g, sugar: 1g, vitamin a: 379iu, vitamin c: 25mg, calcium: 207mg, iron: 5mg.

54. PESTO SHRIMP AND BROCCOLI FETTUCCINE + WEEKLY MENU

Prep time: 5 mins

Cook time: 20 mins

Total time: 25 mins

Serves:8 (about 2 cups of every)

Ingredients

- 1-pound broccoli florets—7 cups of
- 1¼ cup of prepared basil pesto
- 2 lbs cooked or thawed medium shrimp (peeled and deveined)
- ⅓ cup of grated Parmesan cheese

Instructions

Over high heat, bring a large pot of water to a rolling boil. Cook for 6 minutes after adding the fettuccine. This should take around three minutes. Set aside ½ cup of the cooking liquid for later use. Empty the pasta mixture.

Put the spaghetti and broccoli back in the saucepan and reduce the heat. Add shrimp and pesto and stir. Cook, tossing often, for approximately 2 minutes or until thoroughly cooked. If more cooking liquid is needed to get the proper smoothness, add 1 tablespoon. Serve immediately after sprinkling with Parmesan cheese.

Nutrition Information

Serving size: around two cups of 489 calories, 20.8 fat, 48.5 carbs, 3.4 sugar, 942 Sodium, 4 Fiber, 28.8 protein, 138 mg of cholesterol.

55. CREAMY GARLIC BUTTER TUSCAN SCALLOPS

PREP: 10 MINUTES

COOK: 15 MINUTES

TOTAL: 25 MINUTES

INGREDIENTS

- 28 Ounces (800 g) scallops
- 2 tsp salted butter
- 4 cloves garlic, finely diced
- 1 small yellow onion, diced
- 1/2 cup of white wine (OPTIONAL)
- 5 Ounces (150 g) of sun-dried tomato strips in oil that have been jarred and drained; save aside 1 tsp of the oil to be used in cooking
- 1 and a quarter cup of heavy cream (or half and half) NOTES
- Salt and Pepper, as need
- 3 cups of cleaned baby spinach leave
- Grated fresh Parmesan cheese, half a cup
- 2 tsp dried Italian herbs
- 1 tbsp fresh parsley, chopped

INSTRUCTIONS

Dry the scallops completely with paper towels.

Shimmer the olive oil in a large pan set over medium-high heat until it bubbles. Work in batches if necessary, and add the scallops to the pan in a single layer without packing it too full.

When the golden crust forms beneath, season with salt and Pepper as needed, fry for two minutes on one side, then turn and continue cooking for another two minutes or until the food is crisp, lightly browned, and cooked through (opaque). Take out of the skillet and place on a platter.

In the pan, melt the butter. Saute onion for 4 minutes or until it becomes tender. Add the garlic and boil until fragrant, approximately 30 seconds. Add white wine now and let it decrease by half, scraping any crumbs from the pan's bottom. Add sun-dried tomatoes and simmer for one to two minutes to unleash their flavors.

Turn the heat down to low-medium, mix in the heavy cream (or half-and-half), and simmer gently for a few minutes.

Add the parmesan cheese after allowing the spinach to wilt in the sauce. Simmer the sauce for one more minute to let the cheese melt into it.

After thoroughly stirring the herbs, please turn off the heat and add the scallops and their juices to the pan. Before serving, gently stir everything together.

Serve with steamed vegetables, pasta, rice, zoodles, cauliflower rice, or mash.

Have fun!

NUTRITION

516 kcal of calories, 36g of carbohydrates, 38g of protein, and 24g of fat.

56. HEAVENLY HALIBUT

Prep Time: 5 minutes

Cook Time: 15 minutes

Total Time: 20 minutes

Ingredients

- kosher salt and Pepper
- 2 tbsp mayonnaise
- 2 tsp softened butter
- 1.5 tbsp green onions, chopped
- 2 little minced garlic cloves
- ¼ cup of shredded mozzarella cheese
- 2 tsp distilled white vinegar or (if tolerated) lemon juice

Instructions

Set oven temperature to 425°F. Slice the halibut filet into individual servings and sprinkle with kosher salt and Pepper. Mix the mozzarella cheese, green onions, garlic, melted butter, vinegar, and lemon juice. Drizzle over every filet of halibut.

Cook through, approximately 15 minutes, at 425 degrees. Set the broiler to high after removing the halibut. With caution not to overcook, broil the cheese for one minute or until it is gently browned. Warm up and serve.

Nutrition

Serving: 1filet | Calories: 243kcal | Carbohydrates: 2g | Protein: 4g | Fat: 25g | Cholesterol: 47mg | Sodium: 278mg | Sugar: 1g | Calcium: 76mg .

---

57. SALSA SALAD

Preparation and cooking time

Prep:5 mins

Cook:8 mins

Serves 2

Ingredients

- 2 x skinless cod fillets
- 1 lime, zested and juiced
- 1 small mango, peeled, stoned, and chopped (or 2 every, stoned and chopped)
- 1 small avocado, stoned, peeled, and sliced
- ¼ cucumber chopped
- 160g cherry tomatoes, quartered
- 1 red chili, deseeded and chopped
- 2 spring onions, sliced
- handful chopped coriander

Method

Set the oven's temperature to gas 6 and 200°C (or 180°C for fans). Transfer the fish to a shallow ovenproof dish, cover it with half of the lime juice and a little zest, and sprinkle some black pepper. Fish should flake easily but still be juicy after 8 minutes in the oven.

Meanwhile, properly combine the other ingredients, zest, and lime juice in a dish. Transfer to plates, mounding any remaining dish juices on the fish.

58. ONE-PAN SALMON WITH ROAST ASPARAGUS

Prep:20 mins

Cook:50 mins

Serves 2

Ingredients

- 400g new potato, halved if large
- 2 tbsp olive oil
- 8 asparagus spears, trimmed and halved
- 2 handfuls cherry tomatoes
- 1 tbsp balsamic vinegar
- 2 salmon fillets, about 140g/5Ounces every
- handful basil leaves

Method

Set the oven's temperature to 220°C, fan 200°C, and gas 7. After tossing the potatoes with a tbsp of olive oil in an ovenproof dish, bake for 20 minutes or until they brown. Add the asparagus to the potatoes and toss again; bake for fifteen minutes.

Add the cherry tomatoes and vinegar, then tuck the salmon between the veggies. Once the salmon is done, drizzle it with the remaining oil and put it back in the oven for another ten to fifteen minutes. After adding the basil leaves, serve right away, being sure to remove everything from the dish.

Nutrition: per servingHighlightNutrientUnitkcal483 , fat25 g , saturates fat 4g , carbs34g , sugars6g , fibre3g , protein33g , low insalt0.24g .

59. ROASTED SALMON WITH YOGURT DILL SAUCE

Prep Time: 15 mins

Cook Time: 15 mins

Total Time: 30 mins

Yield: 4

INGREDIENTS

- 4 portions of salmon fillets
- 1 Tbsp olive oil
- salt and ground black Pepper

Sauce:

- 3/4 – 1 cup of Greek yogurt
- 1 Tbsp lemon juice
- 1 Tbsp fresh dill, minced
- 1/2 Tbsp fresh chives, minced
- 1 garlic clove
- salt, ground black Pepper, as needed

INSTRUCTIONS

They prepare the yogurt sauce and put it in the fridge while the fish is baking.

Mix the yogurt, chives, dill, and lemon juice. I prefer to crush the garlic lightly, put it into the sauce, and then take it out before serving. This will give the sauce a hint of garlic flavor without making it taste too strong. If you like a more robust garlic flavor, you may also chop the garlic or grate it using a Microplane. As needed, add salt and ground black Pepper for seasoning. Minced capers are a fantastic addition to this sauce.

Set the oven's temperature to 500 degrees Fahrenheit. Turn the oven on to heat and put in a rimmed baking sheet.

Meanwhile, coat every salmon fillet with oil and sprinkle with salt and Pepper.

After the baking sheet has been in the oven for about ten minutes and the stove has reached 500 degrees, remove the baking sheet and lay the salmon, skin side down, on the extremely hot sheet. The skin will immediately begin to sear, and you will hear it sizzle.

Once the oven has warmed, put the fish inside. The fish should be roasted for 12 to 15 minutes at 250 degrees.

Serve the yogurt sauce beside the fish.

CHAPTER SEVEN: POULTRY

60. CHICKEN SALAD WITH APPLES

SERVINGS 1 cup of every

COOK 15 minutes

TOTAL 15 minutes

INGREDIENTS

- 3 cups of chopped cooked chicken
- One apple (1.5 cup of chopped)
- 1/4 cup of diced red onion
- 1/4 cup of dried cranberries
- 1/3 cup of mayonnaise
- 1/3 cup of plain yogurt
- 1 Tbsp Dijon mustard
- 1 Tbsp red wine vinegar
- 1/4 tsp salt
- 1/4 tsp freshly cracked black pepper

INSTRUCTIONS

Cut the apple and the cooked chicken into tiny pieces. Dice the red onion finely.

Put the chicken, apple, onion, and dried cranberries in a big bowl.

Mix the yogurt, Dijon mustard, red wine vinegar, mayonnaise, salt, and Pepper in a bowl. Blend until a smooth consistency is achieved.

Mix everything after adding the dressing to the salad components in the bowl to ensure it is all coated. Before you're ready to eat, serve immediately or store in the refrigerator.

NUTRITION

Serving: 1Serving Calories: 367kcal, Carbohydrates: 15g, Protein: 34g, Fat: 19g, Sodium: 395mg, Fiber: 2g.

61. CHICKEN CLUB MASON JAR SALADS

prep time: 10 minutes

cook time: 35 minutes

Ingredients

- Chicken
- 1.5 lb chicken breast, four pieces
- 1 tsp paprika
- 1 tsp garlic powder
- 1 tsp onion powder
- 1 tsp coriander
- 1/2 tsp ground mustard
- 1 tsp kosher salt

Dressing

- 1/2 cup of nonfat, plain Greek yogurt
- 1/3 tbsp honey
- 1 tbsp Dijon mustard
- 1 tbsp apple cider vinegar
- Salad Components
- 2 hearts of romaine
- 2 scallions
- 1 pint cherry tomatoes
- 1/2 red onion, chopped

- 8 slices center cut bacon
- optional: avocado, not included in nutritional information

Instructions

Set the oven temperature to 400°F.

Place foil on a baking sheet and place a wire rack on top.

Mix up the chicken spice mixture and coat every chicken breast thoroughly.

Turn the heat up to medium-high in a grill pan. Use olive oil spray to coat the grill pan. You may utilize the barbecue as well.

Cook the chicken until it's well done; depending on how thick the chicken is, this may take different amounts of time; for my complete chicken breasts, it took approximately 25 to 30 minutes. Take it off the grill and place it on a cooling rack.

While the chicken cooks, arrange the bacon strips on the wire rack and fry them.

Cook till crispy to your taste, 25 to 30 minutes.

Mix the ingredients for the dressing and reserve.

Chop the chicken when it cools. Chop the scallions and the red onion. Chop the lettuce coarsely.

The salad components are arranged in a mason jar: one cup of chicken, two bacon pieces, red onion, scallions, cherry tomatoes, and lettuce.

Present the dressing as a side dish. Serve every salad with a generous 2 tbsp.

Nutrition

Serving size: one Mason jar salad with two tbsp of dressing; Calories: 332 kcal; Carbohydrates: 15g; Protein: 46g; Fat: 10g; Cholesterol: 110 mg; Sodium: 1091 mg; Potassium: 1128 mg; Fiber: 3g; Sugar: 10g; Calcium: 82 mg; Iron: 2 mg.

62. CHICKEN PESTO WRAPS

PREP: 15minutes

COOK: 5minutes

SERVINGS: 4 wraps

Ingredients

- 2 cups of cooked chicken *see notes
- ⅓ cup of pesto, *add more as needed
- 3 Tbsp grated Parmesan, optional
- 4 wraps
- 4 cups of romaine, shredded
- 1 cup of cherry tomatoes, sliced

Caesar Dressing

- ½ cup of mayo, *see notes
- 2 Tbsp olive oil
- 3 Tbsp fresh lemon juice
- ¼ cup of Parmesan, grated
- 2 garlic cloves
- 1 ½ Tbsp capers and brine
- 2 tsp Dijon mustard
- 2 tsp Worcestershire sauce
- ¼ tsp salt
- ¼ tsp fresh cracked pepper

Instructions

Remove from the heat and chop the cooked chicken into bite-sized pieces. If you are preparing Spinach Walnut Pesto, have the pesto ready. Put aside. Chop the tomatoes and shred the romaine; leave aside.

Put the ingredients for the dressing in a little food processor or blender. Mix thoroughly. Now is the perfect moment as you need the dressing and add extra salt if desired!

Mix the romaine and tomatoes with half the dressing in a medium-sized bowl. Make sure everything is thoroughly mixed and covered.

Mix the chopped chicken with the pesto dressing in a big basin. Make sure the chicken has an even coating of the delectable pesto by thoroughly mixing.

Get the wrap ready. Fill the middle of the wrap with the salad mixture (avoid packing the wrap too full, or it may come apart). Then top with a heaping helping of the pesto chicken. You may use the remaining dressing for dipping or add more Parmesan and dressing if you'd like.

Recline the wrap into a burrito. Eat the wrap immediately or reheat it in a hot pan by spritzing it with oil, putting it on medium heat, and toasting it for two to three minutes on every side.

Nutrition

SERVING: 1 wrap; 583 kcal; 21g of carbohydrates; 24g of protein; 45g of fat; 71 mg of cholesterol; 970 mg of sodium; 342 mg of potassium; 2g of fiber; 3g of sugar; 155 mg of calcium; and 3 mg of iron.

63. MEDITERRANEAN CHICKEN WRAP

prep time: 20 MINUTES

cook time: 10 MINUTES

total time: 30 MINUTES

yield: 3-4

INGREDIENTS

- 1 1/2 lbs / 650g chicken breast, skinless, boneless
- 3 garlic cloves, minced
- 1 tsp chili flakes
- 1 tsp ground black pepper
- 1 1/2 tsp mint, dried
- 1/2 cup of yogurt
- 1/2 tsp dill, dried or 1 tbsp fresh
- salt and Pepper as needed
- hummus
- 1 cup of chopped Cabbage
- everyday salad
- cooked broccoli
- 3-4 tortillas

INSTRUCTIONS

Prepare the salad by chopping the veggies.
To make the garlicky yogurt sauce, blend 1 clove of garlic, dill, and a little salt in a blender.
Cut the chicken into tiny pieces and fry it over medium-high heat in a nonstick pan with 1 tbsp of olive oil. Once the chicken is covered, add the dried mint, black Pepper, chili flakes, and two cloves of garlic and stir. Cook until the chicken is golden brown, 8 to 10 minutes.

Put the wraps together: Add as much as you would like...Place the chopped lettuce or cabbage, chicken, cooked broccoli (if using), tzatziki, hummus, and some salad in the center of every tortilla. Roll up like a tortilla and eat right away.

NUTRITION INFORMATION

Yield4Serving Size1Amount Per ServingCalories488, Total Fat11g, Cholesterol140mg, Sodium511mg, Carbohydrates35g, Fiber4gSugar3g, Protein58g .

64.OVEN CHICKEN KABOBS

Prep Time: 15 minutes

Cook Time: 20 minutes

Total Time: 35minutes

Servings: 4 servings

Ingredients

- 2 tbsp olive oil
- ½ tsp sea salt
- ¼ tsp black Pepper
- 1 tsp garlic powder
- 1 tsp onion powder
- ½ tsp dried thyme
- 2 large chicken breasts (12 ounces every)

Instructions

While preparing the chicken, soak wooden skewers in water for 20 minutes.

Heat the oven to 450°F. Heat the broiler and set a baking sheet with a rim.

Mix the olive oil, onion, garlic, pepper powders, thyme, and salt in a big bowl.

Cut the breasts of the chicken into cubes. Toss the cubes with the seasoned olive oil after adding them to the bowl.

The coated chicken cubes should be skewered.

After the baking sheet is ready, place the kabobs on it. Cover their exposed edges with small pieces of foil to keep wooden skewers from burning. Bake for about 15 minutes or until the kabobs are cooked through.

To broil, turn the oven on. After putting the baking sheet under the broiler for approximately a minute, broil the chicken until it starts to brown. Serve right away.

Nutrition per Serving

A recipe yields 0.25 servings, 250 kcal of calories, 1gram of carbohydrates, 36g of protein, 7g of fat, and 399 mg of sodium.

64. TERIYAKI CHICKEN STIR FRY

Prep: 15minutes

Cook: 20minutes

Total: 35minutes

Servings: 4

Ingredients

- 62 boneless skinless chicken breasts
- 1/2 tsp garlic powder
- Pepper as need
- 3 tbsp cornstarch
- 3 tbsp olive oil divided
- 1/2 medium onion
- 2 cup of broccoli florets
- 1/2 red bell pepper

Sauce:

- 1/2 cup of chicken broth
- 3 tbsp mirin. See note
- 1 tsp of apple cider vinegar (rice vinegar)
- 1/4 cup of brown sugar, packed
- 1 tbsp cornstarch
- 1 tsp finely chopped, fresh ginger
- 2 cloves garlic minced

Instructions

Prepare the ingredients before cooking since recipes come together rapidly once they are underway. Chop the veggies into bite-sized chunks and the broccoli very finely to guarantee they cook all at once.

All the sauce components should be mixed and tossed in a medium-sized bowl.

Slice the chicken into 1-inch chunks and transfer it to a basin. Garlic powder and a little pepper should be added to every slice. Mix everything. Once the cornstarch has been added, mix the chicken to coat it.

Give the pan a few minutes to heat.

For optimal browning, cook the chicken in two batches. Shake off any extra cornstarch before adding half of the chicken to the pan. Simmer for 4 minutes, then turn and cook for 3–4 minutes. To make things easier, I flip using tongs. The chicken has to be well-cooked and browned. Move to a platter. Repeat the process for the second batch after adding the third tbsp of olive oil to the skillet.

Add a bit (approximately a tsp) of olive oil to the pan if it feels dry before adding the onions. Cook, stirring occasionally, for 1 minute.

Cook the broccoli and peppers for three minutes, stirring often, after adding them. Vegetables ought to be crisp-tender. If you would want them softer, cook for a bit longer.

Return the chicken to the pan and toss in the sauce, giving it one more fast whisk before adding it. Stir continuously to ensure that everything is coated while you let it bubble for less than a minute until it thickens. Serve the pan right away after turning off the heat.

Nutrition

360 kcal, 33g of carbs, 27g of protein, 14g of fat, 72 mg of cholesterol, 860 mg of sodium, 674 mg of potassium, 2g of fiber, 19g of sugar, 44 mg of calcium, and 1 mg of iron.

65. BAKED CHICKEN QUESADILLAS

Total Time: 30 minutes

Yield: 4 servings

INGREDIENTS

- 12 ounces boneless skinless chicken breast (approximately 2 breasts), cut into ½ inch cubes
- 3 tbsp fajita seasoning*
- 1 tbsp avocado oil (or vegetable oil)
- ½ medium onion, diced
- 1 red bell pepper, diced
- 1 green bell pepper, diced
- cooking oil spray (or vegetable oil)
- 4 flour tortillas, 8 inches in diameter
- 1 cup of cheddar cheese, shredded and divided
- ½ cup of Monterey Jack cheese, shredded

For serving (optional):

- guacamole
- pico de gallo
- sour cream

INSTRUCTIONS

Turn the oven on to 425F. A large baking sheet should be lined with parchment paper. Put parchment paper on the bottom of a large baking sheet. Add vegetable oil or cook oil spray on the parchment paper to grease it.

Place the cubed chicken and fajita spice into a large mixing basin. Toss to coat the chicken in spice thoroughly. While the oven heats up, set aside.

Heat the oil in a big skillet over medium heat. Cook the cubed chicken for approximately five minutes or until browned. After the chicken is done, move it to a platter and put it aside.

In a big pan set over medium-high heat, warm the olive oil. Add the red, green, and onion peppers to the same skillet. Sauté for 3–4 minutes or until soft. Once again, add the cooked chicken back to the skillet and mix it in with the vegetables. Take off the heat and place aside.

One by one, spread a quarter of the filling over one side of every tortilla. Add two tbsp of Monterey Jack cheese and a quarter cup of cheddar cheese. Place the tortilla wrap, folded in half, on the baking sheet that has been prepared. To ensure that the top of the tortilla adheres to the mixture, gently push it down with the back of a flat spatula.

Continue with the final three tortillas.

To help the tortillas crisp up, lightly mist the top of the folded tortillas with additional cooking spray oil or brush oil.

After placing the baking sheet on the center rack of the oven, bake it for fifteen minutes or until the cheese has melted and the surface is crispy and golden brown. Use the back of a spatula or spoon to gently push the tortilla tops back down if you detect them flipping up while baking.

Cut each tortilla into four pieces, then top with guacamole, salsa, and sour cream.

Nutrition

Total Fat 28.4g, Cholesterol 109.4mg, Sodium 1275.2mg, Total Carbohydrate 34.6g, Sugars 3.5g, Protein 36.1g.

57. LEMON PEPPER CHICKEN

prep time: 15 MINUTES

cook time: 30 MINUTES

total time: 45 MINUTES

SERVINGS: 4 PEOPLE

Ingredients
Sauce

- 2 cups of chicken broth
- 1 chicken bouillon cube
- 3 tbsp heavy cream
- 1 tbsp honey
- ½ tsp brown sugar
- 1 tsp EVERY: mustard powder, parsley, oregano
- 1/8 tsp coarse black pepper

Chicken

- 2 large boneless skinless chicken breasts
- 2 tsp Lemon Pepper Seasoning, see notes
- ¼ cup of flour
- 1-2 tbsp olive oil

Other

- ½ cup of dry white wine see notes
- 3 tbsp butter
- 3 cloves garlic, minced
- 3 tbsp flour
- 1/3 cup of Parmesan cheese, grated

- 2 tbsp lemon juice
- 1 lemon, cut into wedges
- Freshly cracked pepper for serving

Instructions
Work

In a large measuring cup with a spout, mix the sauce ingredients and put aside. Before starting, measure out the remaining ingredients.

Prepare the chicken.
To cut the chicken into two or three thinner slices, cut it in half lengthwise. Place a plastic wrap over it and pound it with a meat mallet's textured side until it is ½ inch thick.

Use lemon pepper spice on both sides. Dredge in flour and gently stroke it onto every side's surface. It gets a little texture from the flour, keeping it from sticking to the pan. Additionally, it somewhat thickens the sauce towards the end.)

Chicken should have a golden crust after being seared in batches for 4–5 minutes on every side. Arrange.

Make the Sauce
Switch off the heat. After adding the wine, reduce the heat to medium. The sauce will taste better if the bottom and sides of the skillet are cleaned with a silicone spatula, creating a "fond." After around three minutes, decrease by half, bringing to a moderate bubble.

Add the garlic and butter, and sauté for an additional minute.

Little splashes of the chicken broth mixture should be added while stirring constantly. (This is the concoction we mixed in the first prep stage.)

Lower the heat to a low simmer after boiling the sauce. Give it five minutes to reduce and simmer. The sauce will thicken and concentrate during this time, and the flavors will blend.

Turn down the heat. Add the Parmesan cheese gradually and whisk constantly until it melts and blends well. Stir in the lemon juice gradually.

Spoon sauce over chicken and return it to the pan. Cover and boil for 4 minutes to reduce. Simmer the fresh lemon wedges in the pan for Another minute after adding them. Take off the heat. After adding some parsley and freshly ground pepper, serve!

Nutrition

345 calories, 18g of protein, 21g of fat, 81mg of cholesterol, 961mg of sodium, 382mg of potassium, 2g of fiber, 7g of sugar, 123mg of calcium, and 2 mg of iron.

58. SHEET PAN BALSAMIC CHICKEN & BRUSSEL SPROUTS

prep time: 10MINUTES

cook time: 20MINUTES

total time: 30MINUTES

yield: 4

INGREDIENTS

- 1 and a half pounds of bite-sized chicken breast
- 1 pound of Brussels sprouts, quartered if big.
- A 1/4 cup of balsamic vinegar
- Powdered garlic, one tsp

- 2 tsp avocado or olive oil
- 1 tsp dried basil
- As needed, add up to 1/2 tbsp of dried oregano
- One tsp sea salt

INSTRUCTIONS

Heat the oven to 400°FLine a silicone baking mat or large baking sheet with parchment paper.

Garlic powder,

Balsamic vinegar, oregano, oil, basil, and sea salt should all be mixed in a big bowl. Mix thoroughly.

Toss in the chopped chicken and Brussels sprouts. Toss in the coat.

Arrange the chicken and Brussels sprouts in a single layer on the baking pan.

The chicken should no longer be pink in the center, and the sprouts tender after 20 minutes in the oven.

Savor it immediately over mashed potatoes or cauliflower rice.

Nutrition

calories: 325 kcal, 14g of carbs, 40g of protein, 12g of fat, 109mg of cholesterol, 1124mg of potassium, 812mg of sodium, 5g of fiber, 5g of sugar, 93mg of calcium, and 3mg of iron.

59. CREAMY MASHED CAULIFLOWER

Prep: 15minutes

Cook: 10minutes

Total: 25minutes

Servings: 6

Ingredients

- 1 kg / 2lb cauliflower florets (Note 1)
- 2 garlic cloves, peeled, whole
- 2 tbsp (30g) unsalted butter
- 1/4 cup of (25g) parmesan cheese, shredded
- 1/4 cup of (55g) sour cream, optional
- 1 - 3 tbsp cooking water
- Salt and pepper, as need

GARNISHES (OPTIONAL):

- Melted butter, parsley, pepper

Instructions

Cut every bigger floret in half or quarters to ensure it is the same size.
Add the cauliflower and garlic in a large saucepan of boiling water and simmer until very tender, about 10 minutes.
Pour some cooking water into a cup.
After thorough draining, put it in a food processor.
Blend the remaining ingredients until smooth, excluding any water at first. Use a handheld blender stick if you don't have a food processor. Use the cooking water set aside to assist purée the meal smoothly and taste.

As needed, adjust the salt and pepper.

Spoon into a serving dish, cover with melted butter, and top with parsley, if you like.

Serve as an accompaniment to any dish that calls for mashed potatoes!

NUTRITION INFORMATION:

Calories:111cal, Carbohydrates:9g, Protein:4g, Fat:7g, Cholesterol:17mg, Sodium:125mg, Potassium:511mg, Fiber:3g, Sugar:3g, Vitamin A:210IU, Vitamin C:80.7mg, Calcium:98mg, Iron:0.7mg .

60. THANKSGIVING LEFTOVER TORTILLA WRAP

PREP: 5minutes

COOK: 5minutes

TOTAL: 10minutes

INGREDIENTS

- 1 large flour tortilla
- 1/4 cup of cranberry sauce
- 1/4 cup of chopped turkey
- 1/4 cup of stuffing
- 3 slices brie

INSTRUCTIONS

Using the same motion as when cutting a tortilla in half, cut the tortilla from the center to the edge, but only halfway.

Transfer the tortilla to a big skillet and set it over medium heat.

Spread the cranberry sauce over one quadrant of the tortilla, starting adjacent to the cut, while the skillet and tortilla heat up. Place the chopped turkey, brie, and stuffing in the quadrants adjacent to the cranberry sauce, brie, and stuffing.

Over the turkey-filled quadrant, fold the tortilla piece dripping with cranberry sauce. Once more, fold it over the brie-covered quadrant. Next, fold it over the stuffing-filled quadrant one last time.

The folded tortilla should be cooked on every side for a few more minutes or until it is crispy and golden. Savor it hot.

NUTRITION

Serving: 1wrapCalories: 600kcal, Carbohydrates: 54g, Protein: 27g, Fat: 31g, Sodium: 1022mg, Fiber: 3g.

61. GROUND TURKEY MEATLOAF WITH BROWN SUGAR GLAZE

PREP TIME: 20 minutes

COOK TIME: 1hour

TOTAL TIME1hour: 20minutes

SERVINGS: 5

INGREDIENTS

- Meatloaf
- 1 1/2 pound ground turkey
- 2 eggs
- Half a cup of onion chopped finely
- 1/2 a cup of carrots, shredded
- 1/4 cup of green bell pepper and diced coarsely
- 1/2 cup of chopped fresh spinach
- Use your preferred bread crumbs or 3/4 cup of quick oats.
- 1/4 cup of ketchup
- 1 tsp The Worcestershire
- 1/2 tsp of garlic powder
- 1/2 tsp Italian spice
- 1/2 tsp dried mustard
- 1 1/2 tsp salt
- 1/2 tsp pepper
- nonstick cooking spray

Brown Sugar Glaze

- 1/4 cup of ketchup
- 1 tbsp Worcestershire

- 2 tbsp brown sugar

INSTRUCTIONS

Warm up the oven to 350°F.

In a large dish, mix all of the meatloaf ingredients. Load a loaf pan generously with nonstick cooking spray on both sides. Evenly disperse everything. Give it thirty minutes in a heated oven.

Meanwhile, mix the glaze components in a small dish.

Cover the meatloaf with glaze after 30 minutes and return to the oven for 30 to 40 minutes. Bake for thirty to forty minutes or until the sauce is thick and the meatloaf is thoroughly cooked. The internal temperature of an instant-read thermometer should be 165 degrees. Before slicing, let the meatloaf rest for ten minutes.

CHAPTER EIGHT: PORK AND BEEF

62. CHEF'S SALAD RECIPE (REMEMBERING NAN)

Prep Time: 15 minutes

Total Time: 15 minutes

Servings: 4 servings

Ingredients

- 8 cups of chopped iceberg lettuce (you may also use red or green leaf lettuce, romaine, or Boston).
- 6 ounces of cooked smoked ham, cut into small cubes (about 1.5 cups)
- After the eggs are removed from their shells, chop or quarter four large hard-boiled eggs.
- 1.5 cups (6 ounces) of cubed cheddar cheese
- ½ round English cucumber, sliced and then cut in half
- A half-cup of cherry or grape tomatoes
- 1 cup of croutons
- salt, as needed (not required)
- freshly ground pepper, as needed (optional)
- Salad Dressing (I like Italian, French, or ranch)

Instructions

Arrange the lettuce, then top with the ham, turkey, eggs, cheddar cheese, cucumber, tomatoes, croutons, and salt and pepper (if used). Toss to combine.

Advice: You can arrange the salad in smaller serving dishes for aesthetic reasons instead of a bigger one, but that's entirely up to you.

To present, separate the salad into individual serving dishes and pour your preferred salad dressing over it to your liking. Have fun!

63. CHEESY HAM & POTATO CASSEROLE

Prep Time: 30 minutes

Cook Time: 45 minutes

Total Time: 1 hour,15 minutes

Yield: serves 10

Ingredients

- 2 pounds (915g) of potatoes (I suggest Yukon Gold or Russet)
- Two cups of diced ham (approximately 300g or eight ounces)
- Shredded sharp white cheddar cheese, 1 and 1/2 cups of (150g or 5.25 ounces), split
- 3 Tbsp (43g) unsalted butter
- Chopped yellow onion, 3/4 cup of (100g) (half of a big onion)
- 3 garlic cloves, minced
- 3/4 tsp salt
- 1/2 a tsp of finely powdered pepper
- 1/2 tsp smoked paprika
- 1/2 a tsp of mustard powder

- 1 tsp dried parsley (or 2 tbsp of fresh minced parsley)
- 1 cup of (24g) all-purpose flour
- 2 cups of (480ml) whole milk
- optional, for garnish: chopped fresh parsley, green onion, chives, or hot sauce

Instructions

After peeling the potatoes, roughly chop them into 3/4-inch pieces. Just over 6 cups of diced potatoes will be left behind. Pour water into a medium saucepan and cover. Heat till boiling. Once boiling, reduce the boiling time to 5–6 minutes. The potatoes should be slightly softened; you don't want them to be extremely delicate and soft. Empty.

Grease a 3- to 4-quart oven-safe dish or a 9-by-13-inch dish. Add the ham, one cup (approximately 100g) of shredded cheese, and the heated, drained potatoes. Toss gently to mix. Put aside.

Heat oven to 375°F (191°C).

In a big skillet or saucepan, Melt the butter over medium heat. Add the garlic and onion, and simmer, stirring periodically, before the onions are tender, about 3 minutes. Add the flour, parsley, ground mustard, smoked paprika, salt, and pepper. Simmer for three to five minutes or until the mixture thickens into a gravy consistency. Stir the flour until the liquid is absorbed. Turn down the heat to low and mix in the milk gently. Take off the heat. Add extra salt, pepper, paprika, mustard, or parsley if preferred.

Cover the ham and potatoes with heated sauce. To coat, gently toss.

Bake for thirty minutes with an aluminum foil cover. Once the cheese has melted and the casserole is bubbling around the edges, remove the aluminum foil, sprinkle the remaining cheese on top, and put it back in the oven for five to ten minutes.

Take out of the oven and top with spicy sauce, chives, green onions, or fresh parsley.

Any leftover food can be kept in the refrigerator for seven days. As desired, reheat. Cover the dish entirely with aluminum foil and bake at 350°F (177°C) for 20 minutes.

64. BAKED PORK CHOPS AND SAUERKRAUT

Prep Time: 10 minutes

Cook Time: 55minutes

Total Time: 1 hour 5minutes

Servings: 4 servings

Ingredients

- One tbsp of olive or avocado oil
- Cut 4 5-ounce pork chops into pieces with a fat thickness of about ½ inch.
- ½ tsp pepper as needed
- ¼ tsp garlic powder
- 1 yellow onion, thinly cut after peeling
- 1 granny smith or gala apple, cored, peeled, and sliced, is fantastic.
- 1 cup of homemade apple cider or store-bought apple cider.
- 2 Tbsp light brown sugar keto, use coconut palm sugar

- 2 pounds sauerkraut in a bag and drained.

Instructions

Sauerkraut and Baked Pork Chops
Set the oven's temperature to 350.
Both sides of the pork chops have been seasoned with garlic powder and black pepper.
Transfer the avocado oil to an ovenproof pan and turn the heat medium. The pork chops should be browned for four minutes on every side. Put aside.
Sliced onion, diced apple, brown sugar, apple juice, and drained sauerkraut should all be added to the pan and mix.
When the sauerkraut and juices are all over the brown pork chops, add them and stir.
Bake the skillet for at least 45 to 60 minutes with a cover or foil on top. The pork chops have to be soft and devoid of pink hue. A temperature of 145 degrees is ideal for pork. When ready to dine, serve right away or chill, then reheat.

Nutrition

Serving: 1chop | Calories: 212kcal | Carbohydrates: 20g | Protein: 15g | Fat: 8g |Cholesterol: 39mg | Sodium: 372mg | Potassium: 333mg | Fiber: 2g | Sugar: 18g |Calcium: 40mg | Iron: 0.7mg.

65. PULLED PORK SWEET POTATO SANDWICH

PREP TIME: 10 minutes

COOK TIME: 15 minutes

TOTAL TIME: 25 minutes

SERVINGS: 12 Servings

INGREDIENTS

- Pulled Pork Sweet Potatoes:
- 3 large Sweet Potatoes
- 1 White Onion diced
- 2 tsp Garlic Powder
- 1 pinch of Fresh Ground Pepper
- 1 pinch of Sea Salt
- 2 Tbsp Vegetable Broth

BBQ Sauce:

- 15 ounces of Organic Tomato Sauce
- 1 Chipotle Pepper in Adobo Sauce
- 2 Tbsp Grape Jelly
- 2 Tbsp Apple Cider Vinegar
- Other Ingredients
- 12 whole grain buns
- 1 recipe of pineapple coleslaw

INSTRUCTIONS

Pulled pork with sweet potatoes

Peel and shred three big sweet potatoes using the shredding blade of a food processor.

Cut the onions into thin pieces.
Add the onions and sweet potatoes that have been shredded to a big bowl.
For seasoning, add garlic powder, salt, and pepper.
Pour in one or two Tbsp of veggie broth.

NUTRITION

Calories: 152kcal, Carbohydrates: 35g, Protein: 3g, Fat: 0.3g, Sodium: 422mg, Potassium: 663mg, Fiber: 6g, Sugar: 12g, Vitamin A: 16469IU, Vitamin C: 10mg, Calcium: 60mg, Iron: 2mg.

66. MEAT LOVER'S CROCK POT CHILI

Prep Time: 20 minutes

Cook Time: 6hours

Total Time: 6 hours 20minutes

Servings: 12 -10

INGREDIENTS

- 1 lb Wright® Brand Bacon chopped
- 1 lb Sausage
- 1 lb Ground Beef
- 2 chopped sweet onions
- 4 cloves of minced garlic
- 3.5 cups of beef broth, adjusted for the desired thickness of chili
- Don't drain 28 Ounces
- can of whole tomatoes
- Don't drain the 15-ounce can of whole tomatoes.

- Do not drain
- two cans of white chili beans with sauce.
- 15-Ounces Tomato Sauce Can
- 1 8 Ounces Can Tomato Sauce
- 3.5 Tbsp of Chili Powder is excellent

Instructions

Cook the bacon over medium heat before it begins to crisp up. After draining, set aside 1 Tbsp of the grease and save the remainder for subsequent uses.

Sauté your onion and garlic in 1 T of bacon fat in the same pan until the onions are transparent.

Meanwhile, sauté the ground beef and sausage in a separate pan until they are thoroughly cooked, then drain.

Mix all ingredients, excluding garnish, in a slow cooker. (Note: For garnish, you should save 1/2 cup of bacon).

Before cooking, slightly split apart the entire tomatoes with a wooden spoon.

Cook for 6 to 8 hours on low, stirring now and again.

Add more bacon, cheese, sour cream, cooked macaroni noodles, and chopped green onion as garnish.

Nutrition

450 kcal of calories, 14g of carbohydrates, 28g of protein, 32g of fat, 91mg of cholesterol, 1638mg of sodium, 923mg of potassium, 3g of fiber, 8g of sugar, 78mg of calcium, and 3.8 mg of iron.

67. BASIL MEATBALLS

PREP 15minutes

COOK 30minutes

TOTAL 45minutes

INGREDIENTS
Baked Italian Meatballs:

- 1 cup of Parmesan grated
- 3 cloves garlic smashed
- Fresh 20 big basil leaves are usually the best.
- 1 1/2 pounds of ground beef grass-fed is recommended
- 1 pound of pork ground
- 1 cup of panko bread crumbs
- 1 tbsp dried oregano
- 1 tsp ground pepper
- 1/2 tsp red pepper flakes
- 1 large egg, slightly beaten
- 1 tsp kosher salt

Spaghetti and Meatballs:

- 2 28-ounce jars of marinara sauce
- 1 pound pasta

INSTRUCTIONS
To make the meatballs:

Set oven temperature to 400°F. Put parchment paper on a big baking sheet with a rim. Alternatively, because air contact will allow the meatballs' bottoms to brown uniformly, you may make even more excellent meatballs by placing an oven-safe baking rack on top of a baking sheet.

The Parmesan, basil leaves, garlic, and red onion should all be appropriately mixed in a food processor. It ought to be like a thick pesto.

Use your hands to thoroughly mix the remaining ingredients—aside from the salt—in a large dish with the basil mixture. Avoid overmixing. After mixing, add the salt and stir just until it is evenly distributed.

Shape the meatball mixture into tiny, tbsp-sized balls. I like to use a cookie dough scoop to get them all the same size.

Arrange on the baking sheet in a uniform layer, about 0.5 inches apart. I had room for forty on a single baking sheet. Two batches of cooking will likely be required.

Cook 30 to 35 minutes until beautifully browned in a heated oven on a prepared baking sheet. If you need to find out whether the meatballs are done, they should be 160 degrees Fahrenheit.

To make spaghetti and meatballs:

To prepare spaghetti with meatballs, put the necessary number of meatballs into a big saucepan of simmering sauce. Cook until meatballs and sauce are well heated.

NUTRITION

539 kcal, 40g of carbohydrates, 31g of protein, 27g of fat, 109mg of cholesterol, 522mg of sodium, 470mg of potassium, 2g of fiber, 2g of sugar, 174mg of calcium, and 3mg of iron.

68. UNSTUFFED PEPPERS

PREP TIME:10minutes

COOK TIME:1hour

TOTAL TIME1hour:10minutes

SERVINGS:4 servings

INGREDIENTS

- 1 pound lean ground beef
- 2 green bell peppers chopped
- 1 small onion chopped
- 1 tbsp olive oil
- 2 garlic cloves minced
- 2 tsp oregano
- 1 tsp salt
- ½ tsp black pepper
- 2 tbsp tomato paste
- ½ cup of grain white rice
- 15 ounce canned diced tomatoes
- ½ cup of water
- ½ cup of shredded cheddar cheese
- ¼ cup of chopped parsley

INSTRUCTIONS

In a large pot set over medium heat, warm the olive oil. Add ground meat, onions, garlic, green peppers, oregano, salt, and pepper. Simmer for 7 to 10 minutes or until beef is browned.

After adding the tomato paste, cook for two to three minutes or until aromatic and thoroughly mixed. Stir together the rice, water, and diced tomatoes. Put the olive oil into a big saucepan over medium heat. Add ground meat, onions, green peppers, garlic, oregano, salt, and pepper. Simmer until meat is browned, 7 to 10 minutes.

Please remove the heat and cover it for another five to ten minutes. Use a fork to fluff the rice and separate it.

Serve in dishes with parsley and cheddar cheese grated on top.

NUTRITION

333kcal, 27g of carbohydrates, 31g of protein, 11g of fat, 85mg of cholesterol, 815mg of sodium, 701mg of potassium, 3g of fiber, 4g of sugar, 160mg of calcium, and 4mg of iron.

---

69. BUNLESS BURGER

Prep Time: 15 minutes

Cook Time: 5minutes

Total Time: 20 minutes

Servings: 2 servings

Ingredients

- 4 (¼ lb) ground beef patties
- ½ tsp Diamond Crystal kosher salt
- ½ tsp black pepper
- 2 tsp Dijon mustard
- 4 lettuce leaves
- 2 thick tomato slices
- 2 red onion slices
- 2 slices sharp cheddar

Instructions

Add salt and pepper to the meat patties for seasoning. Cook them to your preferred doneness on a medium-high heat cast iron skillet. I fry them for three minutes on every side at medium heat. Grilling is another option.

After transferring the cooked patties to a platter, give them five minutes to rest with a loose foil cover.

As the meat is resting, put the other ingredients together.

To put together the "sandwiches," take out two plates. Put one cooked burger onto every platter. Spread mayo on it if you'd like, but I like mustard. Layer the lettuce, onion, tomato, and cheese over the mustard, then place another cooked burger on top. Serve right away and provide extra napkins.

Nutrition per Serving

Serving: 1 burger - 2 patties with fillings | Calories: 610kcal | Carbohydrates: 3g | Protein: 49g | Fat : 43g | Sodium: 729mg.

70. MINI TACOS

Prep: 10minutes

Cook: 20minutes

Total: 30minutes

Servings: 30 tacos

Ingredients

- 1 pound lean ground beef or boneless, skinless chicken breast, finely chopped.
- 1 tbsp of spice for tacos.
- 30 tortillas (corn or wheat)
- 3 tbsp of vegetable oil, canola oil, or cooking spray.
- 8 ounces cheese Jack, Cheddar, Cojito or American, shredded

Instructions

Turn the oven on to 425°F.

In a pan over medium heat, brown the meat, breaking it up with a spatula or potato masher. After adding taco spice, cook until the pink color disappears. Take off the heat.

Grind corn tortillas or flour using a 3-inch cookie or biscuit cutter. Before cutting corn tortillas, reheat them in the microwave for 30 seconds while holding moist paper towels or a damp towel between them.

Place tortillas on a baking sheet covered with parchment paper after brushing every side with oil.

Stuff with meat or chicken and grated cheese.

For two minutes, bake. Take out of the oven and use tongs or a metal spatula to fold in half. To fold, press.

For 8 to 10 minutes, bake until golden brown on the edges.

Take it out of the oven and top it with your preferred toppings.

72. ROAST BEEF WRAPS

PREP TIME: 10 minutes

TOTAL TIME: 10 minutes

SERVINGS: 4 wraps

INGREDIENTS

- Horseradish Cream Sauce
- ¼ cup of nonfat Greek yogurt
- 2 Tbsp mayonnaise
- ⅛ tsp grated horseradish
- For the roast beef Wrap
- 4 12" flour tortillas
- ¾ pound deli roast beef
- ½ cup of shredded cheddar cheese
- lettuce leaves

INSTRUCTIONS

Tortillas that are just heated enough to be flexible.
Spread the horseradish cream sauce over a flat surface. Top every wrap with sliced roast meat, cheese, and lettuce.
Fold the sides in, then wrap up like a burrito until it's closed.

NUTRITION

Serving: 1grams Calories: 692 kcal, Carbohydrates: 85g, Protein: 33g, Fat: 23g, Saturated Fat: 7g.

CHAPTER NINE: DESSERT

73. FRESH PEVERY COBBLER

Prep Time: 30 minutes

Cook Time: 45 minutes

Total Time: 1 hour, 20 minutes

Yield: serves 10-12

Ingredients
Pevery Filling

- 3.5–4 pounds of fresh every, chopped into 1-1.5-inch pieces after peeling (about 10 cups of or 1.5kg)
- 1/4 cup of (50g) packed light or dark brown sugar
- 1 Tbsp (7g) cornstarch
- 15ml or 1 tbsp of lemon juice
- 1 tsp pure vanilla extract
- 1/2 tsp ground cinnamon
- 1/8 tsp ground nutmeg
- 1/8 tsp ground ginger
- 1/8 tsp salt

Biscuit Topping

- 2 cups of (250g) all-purpose flour (spooned & leveled)
- 1/2 cup of (100g) granulated sugar
- 1 and 1/2 tsp baking powder
- 1/4 tsp baking soda
- 1/2 tsp salt
- 1/2 cup of (8 Tbsp; 113g) unsalted butter, cold and cubed
- 1/2 cup of (120ml) buttermilk, cold*

- 1 giant egg, beaten with one tbsp (15 ml) of milk or buttermilk, is the egg wash.
- optional: 2 Tbsp (25g) granulated sugar mixed with 1/2 tsp ground cinnamon

Instructions

Turn the oven on to 350°F, or 177°C. Grease a 9 x 13-inch baking pan very lightly. You may use any 3- to 4-quart baking dish.

Regarding the filling: Mix all the filling ingredients into the baking pan. For ten minutes, bake. Take out of the oven and place aside while you make the topping. Turn the oven on again.

Mix the flour, baking powder, sugar, baking soda, and salt for the garnish in a large basin. Add the cold butter and chop it into coarse, pea-sized crumbs with two forks or a pastry cutter. Using a pastry cutter expedites and simplifies this procedure! Another option is to use a food processor. Add the buttermilk and stir with a gentle hand until well blended. After everything is well incorporated, the dough should be somewhat sticky; if it's too dry, add one more tbsp of buttermilk.

Put the cobbler together: Scoop out dough and carefully press it onto a flat surface. Cover the whole surface of the heated pevery filling with dough. Flatten the dough into slices and cover most pieces; no specific technique is involved.

Add egg wash to the biscuit dough's top, and if desired, sprinkle with cinnamon and sugar.

Bake for 40 to 50 minutes, until the very filling bubbles around the edges and the biscuit topping is golden brown. The dish is done if a toothpick inserted into the biscuit topping comes out clean.

Place the pan on a wire rack after removing the cobbler from the oven. Before serving, let cool for five minutes. Serve warm with ice cream, vanilla, or whipped cream.

The remaining food can be covered and refrigerated for up to five days.

74. SWEDISH APPLE PIE (EASY CRUSTLESS APPLE PIE)

Prep Time: 15 minutes

Cook Time: 50 minutes

Total Time: 1 hour 4minutes

Servings: 12

Ingredients

- 2 pounds of peeled, cored, and sliced apples into ½-inch thick pieces
- ¼ cup of sugar
- 1 tbsp freshly squeezed lemon juice
- 2 tsp finely ground cinnamon
- ½ tsp ground cardamom
- 1 cup of flour
- ¾ cup of packed light brown sugar

cup of dense brown sugar

- ½ a tsp of salt
- ½ tsp of baking powder
- 1 big egg

- 1 tsp vanilla essence
- ½ cup of unsalted butter, heated and chilled, + more to line the pie dish
- Turbinado sugar to use as a garnish

Instructions

Set oven temperature to 350 degrees. Set aside a 9-inch deep dish pie pan greased with butter.

Mix the apples, sugar, lemon juice, cinnamon, cardamom, and salt in a big bowl. Spoon into the pie pan that has been ready.

Whisk the flour, baking powder, and salt; mark for later. Whisk together the eggs, vanilla, brown sugar, and melted butter in a large bowl. Whisk to mix thoroughly. Using a rubber spatula, dry the liquid components.

After equally distributing the batter over the apples, top with turbinado sugar.

Bake for approximately fifty minutes until the apples are bubbling around the edges and the top is golden brown. Before serving, let cool.

Nutrition

221 kcal of calories, 37g of carbohydrates, 2g of protein, 8g of fat, 34 mg of cholesterol, 126mg of sodium, 122mg of potassium, 2g of fiber, 25g of sugar, 36mg of calcium, and 1mg of iron.

75. KETO PEANUT BUTTER BALLS

Prep Time: 30 minutes

Freezing Time: 1hour

Total Time: 30 minutes

Servings: 24 truffles

Ingredients

- Peanut Butter Cookie Dough:
- 5 tbsp butter
- ¼ cup of peanut butter
- ⅓ cup of powdered Swerve Sweetener
- ½ tsp vanilla extract
- ¾ cup of lightly roasted peanut flour
- Chocolate Coating:
- 3 ounces sugar-free dark chocolate chopped
- ½ ounce cocoa butter or ½ tbsp coconut oil
- 2 tbsp finely chopped salted peanuts optional

Instructions
Cookie Dough
Spread parchment or waxed paper on a large baking sheet.
In a large microwave-safe dish, mix the butter and peanut butter and microwave until melted. After it's smooth, mix in the sweetener and vanilla extract

Stir in the peanut flour just until a stiff dough forms. Add extra flour if the dough looks too sticky to roll into balls.
Place the 1-inch rolled dough balls on the baking sheet that has been heated. Freeze for one hour or until solid.

Milk Chocolate Coverage

Put the chocolate and cocoa butter into a heat-resistant dish and place it over a pan of water that is just simmering. Mix until smooth and melted.

With a fork, roll the frozen peanut butter balls around in the chocolate. To get rid of extra chocolate, lift it out and tap the fork firmly on the bowl's side.

When making buckeyes, dunk the peanut butter balls in the chocolate and twirl with a small stick to coat. Just the ball's topmost top should remain uncoated.

Reposition on the baking sheet and, if desired, top with chopped peanuts. If the dough balls are frozen, the chocolate will solidify rapidly, so immediately sprinkle every truffle after dipping it in chocolate.

Nutrition Facts
Keto Peanut Butter Balls

Amount Per Serving (2 truffles)

Calories 131Calories from Fat 104, Fat 11.6g, Carbohydrates 5.2g, Fiber 3.2g, Protein 2.9g.

76. CANNOLI CHEESECAKE STUFFED STRAWBERRIES

Prep Time: 20 minutes

Total Time: 20 minutes

Servings: 16 to 20 strawberries

Ingredients

- 8 ounces cream cheese
- ½ cup of ricotta cheese
- 1 tsp vanilla extract
- ⅔ cup of powdered sugar
- 16-ounce container of strawberries
- Mini chocolate chips for garnish
- Graham cracker crumbs for garnish

Instructions

Beat the cream cheese, ricotta cheese, powdered sugar, and vanilla in a medium-sized bowl. Mix until smooth, about 2 minutes.

The mixture should be refrigerated until ready to fill strawberries.

Strawberries should have their stems removed and sliced across to make them lay flat on a platter. To make room for filling, hollow out or form a cross on the top of a strawberry.

In every strawberry, pipe in a bit of filling. Before serving, top with chocolate chips and graham cracker crumbs.

Nutrition

Serving: 1strawberry | Calories: 91kcal | Carbohydrates: 8g | Protein: 2g | Fat: 6g | Cholesterol: 20mg | Sodium: 52mg | Potassium: 71mg | Fiber: 1g | Sugar: 7g | Calcium: 34mg | Iron: 1mg.

---

77. NO-BAKE CHOCOLATE COCONUT SNOWBALLS

Prep Time: 55 minutes

Cook Time: 3 minutes

Total Time: 1 hour, 30 minutes

Ingredients

- 3 cups of (255g) old-fashioned whole-rolled oats
- 3 cups of (240g) sweetened shredded coconut, divided
- 113g or 1/2 cup of (8 Tbsp) unsalted butter
- 1 cup of (200g) granulated sugar
- 1/2 cup of milk (any milk is OK; I use skim milk)
- 6 Tbsp (32g) unsweetened natural or Dutch-process cocoa powder
- 1/8 tsp salt
- 1 tsp pure vanilla extract

Instructions

Put the oats and one cup of shredded coconut in a big bowl. Set aside. To use with the leftover coconut, save the third step.

Butter, sugar, milk, cocoa, and salt should all be mixed in a big pot and cooked over medium heat. When the butter has melted, stir together and bring to a boil. Boil for one minute without stirring. Please remove the heat, mix the vanilla essence, and cover the oats and coconut. Mix until well blended. For at least 45 minutes and up to two or three days, firmly cover with plastic wrap or aluminum foil and refrigerate.

In the meantime, pulse the remaining coconut to break it up in a food processor. Coating the balls becomes more straightforward when the coconut shreds are smaller and more broken.

Put parchment paper or silicone baking mats in the bottoms of two baking dishes. Additionally, confirm that your refrigerator has adequate space for the baking sheets.

Roll into 1 tbsp balls using a 1-tbsp cookie scoop (or a spoon). The mixture could become sticky as you work, but try your best to roll it into a ball. Place the coconut-rolled balls on the baking sheets. To help it "set," refrigerate for at least 30 to 60 minutes.

Covered snowballs can be kept fresh for three days at room temperature or refrigerated for one week.

78. FRESH MANGO SALSA

Prep Time: 15 mins

Total Time: 15 minutes

Yield: 3 cups of

INGREDIENTS

- 3 ripe mangos, diced
- 1 chopped medium red bell pepper
- ½ cup of chopped red onion
- ¼ cup of packed fresh cilantro leaves, chopped
- 1 jalapeño, seeded and minced
- 1 large lime, juiced (about ¼ cup of lime juice)
- ⅛ to ¼ tsp salt, as needed

INSTRUCTIONS

The prepped mango, bell pepper, onion, cilantro, and jalapeño should all be mixed in a serving dish. Pour one lime juice over it.

Mix the ingredients by stirring them with a big spoon. Add salt as needed and whisk once more. Allow the salsa to rest for at least ten minutes for optimal taste.

79. SUN-DRIED TOMATO PESTO

Prep Time: 5

Total Time: 5 minutes

Yield: 1 1/2 cups of

Ingredients
Regarding the Pesto

- Oil-filled 240 g (8.5 Ounces) jar of sun-dried tomatoes
- one or two cloves of garlic
- Pine nuts, 60 g (1/2 cup of)
- packed cup of (30 g) of fresh basil
- Freshly grated Parmesan cheese, 25 g (1/4 cup)
- When necessary, use olive oil to thin the sauce.
- To Serve (if desired)
- 1 pound (450 g) of rigatoni pasta
- Fresh mozzarella, shredded into bite-sized pieces without salt
- Decorative fresh basil leaves

Instructions

Put some oil and the sun-dried tomatoes in a food processor. Add the Parmesan cheese, garlic, and pine nuts. For flavor, sprinkle in a couple of grinds of black pepper. Process till smooth. When done, it will have a rustic appearance rather than a polished one. To relax the texture taste, add additional olive oil as necessary.

Spoon into an airtight container or basin. Chill for up to four days or until needed.

If you're serving room-temperature pasta, cook, drain, and cool it on a rimmed baking sheet. Disperse it. Add a thin layer of oil.

When ready to add the pesto, let it cool to room temperature. After that, move the mixture to a big bowl, mix in some pesto, top with fresh mozzarella, and sprinkle with basil leaves. Allow to settle at room temperature.

80. PARMESAN CRISPS

Hands-On Time: 5 mins

Total Time: 33 mins

Servings: 11

Ingredients

- 2 ounces grated fresh Parmesan cheese (about 1/2 cup)
- ¼ tsp freshly ground black pepper

Directions

Turn the oven on to 400°F.

Line parchment paper with a large baking sheet. Place tbsp of cheese separated by two inches on the prepared baking sheet. Make every mound a diameter of two inches. Season plenty with pepper. Heat the oven to 400°f for 6-8 minutes or until crisp and golden. On the baking sheet, let cool thoroughly. Remove with a tiny spatula off the baking sheet.

81. HERB AND GARLIC QUINOA

PREP TIME: 2minutes

COOK TIME: 20minutes

TOTAL TIME: 22minutes

SERVINGS: 3

Ingredients

- 1 cup of quinoa
- 2 cups of water
- 2 tsp oil
- ½ tsp salt
- ½ tsp garlic powder
- ½ tsp onion powder
- 1 tsp Italian herb blend

Instructions

Give the quinoa a thorough rinse under cold running water.

All the ingredients should be mixed in a medium and heated until boiling. For approximately ten minutes, or until the quinoa is cooked, reduce heat to medium-low, cover, and simmer.

Please take off the heat and leave it covered for five minutes.

Using a fork, fluff, and serve!

82. MASHED CAULIFLOWER AND POTATOES

Prep Time: 10 minutes

Cook Time: 20 minutes

Total Time: 30 minutes

Servings: 8 people

Ingredients

- Two pounds of russet or yellow potatoes, washed and roughly chopped. Consult the notes.
- Cut 1 medium cauliflower head into individual florets.
- Four cups of stock, either vegetable or poultry. Depending on your taste, you may need less salt if you use Instant Pot
- salt.
- 1 garlic head with the peel removed
- 1 tbsp olive oil
- 4 tbsp butter, more to your liking
- ¾ cup of whole milk, more if desired
- 2 tbsp fresh parsley for serving (optional)
- fresh ground black pepper for Serving

Instructions

For stove-top cooking:

Fill a big saucepan with two pounds of potatoes and one medium head of cauliflower. To cover the veggies, add 4 cups of chicken or vegetable broth. Although you may use water in its place, the broth's flavor is enhanced. Add two cloves of garlic from the already-skinned head of garlic, along with approximately tsp salt, to the saucepan. (Set aside the remaining cloves for roasting.)

When the potatoes are fork-tender, around 20 minutes should pass after bringing them to a boil, covering, and simmering.

While the potatoes and cauliflower are simmering, heat the broiler and position the oven rack one position below the center. Arrange the remaining 7 or 8 garlic cloves on a foil-lined sheet and pour one tbsp of olive oil over them—season with a bit of salt and black pepper. Depending on the oven's heat, place the foil on the rack and bake for 5 to 7 minutes or until the cloves' edges begin to brown. Take great care to ensure the cloves do not burn. Cut the cloves from the oven and chop them until they resemble mashed garlic. Put aside.

After draining, add the potatoes and cauliflower back to the saucepan. Toss in the roasted garlic mash and 4 tsp of butter. Using a potato masher, mash the vegetables before the butter is melted.

After adding ¾ cup of milk, mash the mixture until it reaches the desired consistency. If necessary, add additional milk or butter.

Transfer to a serving plate, whisk, and add more salt as needed. For added appeal, top with a pat of butter, two tablespoons of fresh parsley, and black pepper just before serving.

For Instant Pot or other pressure cooker:

Add potatoes, cauliflower, and two cups of chicken or vegetable broth to the pressure cooker insert. Although you may use water in its place, the broth's flavor is enhanced. Add two cloves of garlic from the already-skinned head of garlic, along with approximately tsp salt, to the saucepan. (Set aside the remaining cloves for roasting.)

Close the cooker's cover, choose Manual mode, and cook for ten minutes at high pressure. (While the potatoes and cauliflower are simmering, prepare the roasted garlic; see the following step.) After the ten minutes, relax the pressure naturally for five minutes before concluding with a brief release. Remove the lid after all pressure has been released and the top is easily turntable.

Heat the broiler and slide an oven rack one position below the center while the potatoes and cauliflower are under pressure. Arrange the remaining 7 or 8 garlic cloves on a foil-covered baking sheet and pour the 1 Tbsp olive oil. Add a tiny tsp of salt and black pepper for seasoning. Depending on the oven's heat, place the foil on the rack and bake for 5 to 7 minutes or until the cloves' edges begin to brown. Take great care to ensure the cloves do not burn. Cut the cloves from the oven and chop them until they resemble mashed garlic. Put aside.

Transfer the potatoes and cauliflower to a large bowl using a slotted spoon. (If you make the recipe dairy-free, use the broth instead of the milk or butter; otherwise, do not pour any leftover broth or water into the dish.)Add the butter and mashed roasted garlic, then use a vegetable masher to mash the potato until the butter is melted.

After adding ¾ cup of milk, mash the mixture until it reaches the desired consistency. If necessary, add additional milk or butter.

As needed, add more salt. Before serving, top with a dollop of butter, fresh parsley, and black pepper for an even more alluring appearance.

Nutrition Facts

Amount Per Serving (1 cup of)

Calories 199Calories from Fat 72, Cholesterol 17mg,
Sodium 558mg2, Potassium 737mg, Carbohydrates 27g, Fiber 2g, Sugar 4g, Protein 4g, Calcium 66mg, Iron 1.4mg.

www.ingramcontent.com/pod-product-compliance
Lightning Source LLC
Chambersburg PA
CBHW071929210526
45479CB00002B/611